EVERYTHING YOU DIDN'T KNOW
ABOUT THE BUSINESS OF MEDICINE

THE
DARK SIDE
OF
MEDICINE

Published by Impact Publishing®, Orlando, FL.

Impact Publishing® is a registered trademark.

Printed in the United States of America.

ISBN: 978-1-7369881-8-3
LCCN: 2022906360

This publication is designed to provide accurate and authoritative information with regard to the subject matter covered. It is sold with the understanding that the publisher is not engaged in rendering legal, accounting, or other professional advice. If legal advice or other expert assistance is required, the services of a competent professional should be sought. The opinions expressed by the authors in this book are not endorsed by Impact Publishing® and are the sole responsibility of the author rendering the opinion.

Most Impact Publishing® titles are available at special quantity discounts for bulk purchases for sales promotions, premiums, fundraising, and educational use. Special versions or book excerpts can also be created to fit specific needs.

For more information, please write:
Impact Publishing®
P.O. Box 950370
Lake Mary, FL 32795
Tel: 1.877.261.4930

EVERYTHING YOU DIDN'T KNOW ABOUT THE BUSINESS OF MEDICINE

THE DARK SIDE OF MEDICINE

By
Dr. Irfan Siddiqui

Impact Publishing®
Lake Mary, Florida

CONTENTS

INTRODUCTION

There are many benefits that come into your life when you're ready to start thinking bigger and beyond the expected.

If you're thinking about entering into the medical industry pipeline—or perhaps you're just about to emerge into the working world—there are other things you'll want to consider as well. Think of the four-burner stove. You can cook your main course on the front burner, but you also have three burners that are not being used. I see future livelihoods as being an opportunity to diversify what you have cooking: perhaps on low, perhaps on simmer, or maybe a big pot on the front. Consider that when you're doing anything as your main course, you still have to consider variable sources of incomes, opportunities. Diversification is key to truly thriving. And the best way to do this is to open up your opportunities and start exploring.

Medical students and industry professionals like myself know and expect that the journey is a long, arduous, and expensive process. The timeframe between when you start medical school and move to your first job in the field could take 8-15 years! But most of us can't put our finances, dreams, and other interests on hold for one or two decades. An 'I'll deal with it later' attitude does not work in this world. Put yourself into a position that, when you look five years ahead, you can be proud and grateful that you made certain choices (even compromises) over time.

This book helps you understand how and why it's important to always think bigger, seeding other opportunities and long-term planning into your goals. Whether you're trading stocks, investing in cryptocurrency, or buying an apartment complex for passive income, it's important to have something else going on – on the side. By sharing my past and present experiences and the wisdom that took me years to gain, I hope to better prepare those who are getting ready to walk a similar path in their future. I want everyone to see there are other areas they can focus on and also find success.

Here's something to consider:

1. What are your goals?
2. Do you view yourself as someone who is going to change the way others think?
3. Do you view yourself as someone who's going to do what it takes to fit in with normative society?

In order to make change you have to think about how you are going to improve or make an impact, but also prepare to go against social norms sometimes. So open up your mind! There's more to life than the medical pipeline that you're getting ready to jump into with excitement and full force. Get ready for your future—not just your career—and start thinking outside the pipeline.

ACKNOWLEDGEMENTS

I have to start at the very beginning...and thank my mom and dad. As the son of these two smart and dynamic individuals, I can see where many of my traits and behaviors come from. For example, my logical reasoning came from my dad, whereas my mom had a special drive that I no doubt inherited—her way of interacting and navigating with the world. Without my parents, I would not be here today, nor would I be the quality of person I am today.

I want to say thank you to Natalie, my spouse, my best friend and life partner. She has been here for me through my ups and downs, and she's pushed me along the way and continues to inspire me daily. I am so grateful for her love and our partnership.

I'd also like to credit two of my mentors: Dr. Joanne Mitchell, the great doctor and director of a medical education program in Michigan, and Dr. Rodney Badger of the University of Utah. Dr. Mitchell guided the first half of my early career, and Dr. Badger the latter half; both gave me so much confidence and opportunities to think outside of the box. I credit them for both granting me liberties to become the physician I am today.

I wanted to write this book for my children so that they and their peers could have a model or some kind of idea, of how to approach the world from a different point of view. Really, it was about changing their thinking. What do we need to do and how can we pivot, change, evolve? The intent of this book was to leave something behind for them to read, whether during the years of publication or twenty years from now. I hope it will open up their thoughts and viewpoints for the future, and remind them to stay curious and open, while also driven to do things their own way.

And, certainly, the audience of this book is worth acknowledging here as well. Perhaps that's you: the intern, the nurse, the resident, the teacher, the fresh-out-of-school physician. When I started writing this book, you were who I had in my mind based on my own journey.

Finally, I want to thank everyone else who has helped me along the way.

SOME FINAL THOUGHTS

Dr. Badger helped me with mindset as well as leadership. He gave me a mindset I'll never forget – You are a lion! The world needs to hear you roar. So with that, I'll end with a call to action: read these words, think about how you might find your own path through, your own successes and futures. Become the best person you can be. Maximize your potential. ROAR!

"It's hard to beat somebody who never gives up."

CHAPTER 1

THE EARLY DAYS

Born and raised in Miami, Florida, a son of immigrants. That's a story like many others, but, I promise, it gets much more interesting from here.

Pakistani culture always emphasizes education. My dad was a civil engineer, and my mom worked for the police department in their Crime Scene Investigation (CSI) unit. Being of Indian-Pakistani culture and the son of two professionals, I was bound to be fast-tracked straight into being both a stellar student and put into some level of extreme prominence in my respective career. It wasn't a suggestion; it was expected – and in some ways, demanded.

When it came time for high school, I went into a magnet program – a school designed to help point students into certain career fields. At this time, being put into the medical program, I had an idea. I wanted to be a doctor; the problem was, I never really felt the drive to get the grades you'd imagine for an up-and-coming student, much to my parents' aggravation. I suppose it goes to show that you'll really do anything to rebel against your parents as a teenager – and I was good at it!

After those years, I moved on to college, of course, where I got into a program where they guaranteed me a seat in their medical school when the time came.

Do you think my hustling stopped when I got to med school, though? Not at all. Time to spin some discs! I was a popular DJ, even using some of my time DJ'ing to mix some of my own music tracks. Interestingly enough, I love...love listening to music, and I wound up becoming a cardiologist, listening to heartbeats all day now.

STUDENT DAZE

The fun fact is that I was never the best student out there. I'm sure this sentiment resonates with most of us. I wasn't the top guy in the class; in fact, I preferred going near the back of the room where I could 'multitask' the entire time. Checking my cell phone, doing other assignments, studying for other tests. We've all been there. The world today is all about multitasking, and we've all been programmed to have ADHD brains with cell phones and video games at our fingertips no matter where we go. And remember, this was a while back, so the problem wasn't as pronounced as it is today!

In the last few years of medical school, though, the goals on my agenda began shifting in my mind like a manic jigsaw puzzle. This activity turned into an aggressive plan-of-attack on my life goals.

"What am I going to do with my life? More importantly, what am I going to do when it comes down to medicine? I'm here; there's no way I can back out now."

That exact thought was one strong enough to freeze me in my tracks. It was time to get everything in order before it was too late. There are plenty of books out there that will tell you that it is 'never too late' – well, for this, it was coming up so fast that the marker for it was blurry in my mind's eye.

- *General Practitioner...*
- *Surgeon...*

- *Orthopedist...*
- *Pediatrician...*

I went through the options one after the other, judging my gut reaction to each, not getting many pings off any of them. It wasn't working out so well.

- *Cardiologist...* A little more excitement there.
- *Interventional Cardiologist...* Bingo. Plenty of training. Three years of internal medicine. Three more years of Cardiology.

'Fantastic...' quipped back my bad internal student voice, '... you're a glutton for punishment.'

A SUPER-SPECIALIST RESIDENCY IS PRETTY EASY, COMPARATIVELY

During this time, you're both learning and studying under the supervision of doctors, getting your 'feet really wet' per se. You're on the floor helping to save lives, but with the safety net of always having a doctor follow up behind you to double-check your work and conference with you about your choices. It's a blissful time. The pressure is on, but it is a simmer compared to the full boil of working solo.

It is also during this time that you're forced to buckle down and select your specialization. This is where you go from a medical student to a future general practitioner, pediatrician, or whatever your choice may be. That's the not-so-easy part.

I've loved doing stuff with my hands my whole life, so all those hobby projects of Legos, widgets, and homemade contraptions I made, being a cardiac interventional cardiologist, where you're putting tiny wires, the size of your hair inside a person, inside an artery, that is, inside your heart, is a very fulfilling and natural fit. I made my choice, and the rest is history.

From there on, you become a 'super-specialist' – one of perhaps a maximum of one hundred graduates each year. For this year, at least the pool of competition was thousands of cardiology resident graduates, factoring myself in.

After graduation, I got recruited straight into a hospital system, the CHS hospital system, a large hospital system, and then packaged off straight to Orlando, Central Florida. My parents lived in South Florida, so I wanted to be close to them; it was a great, non-stressful fit.

At this stage, you're doing the same thing you were doing previously. Still, the difference is that now there's nobody there to back you up – no 'attending physician' to step in. You're on your own, buddy. Welcome to healthcare.

A System Explained

When looking at a large hospital ecosystem, we're all various cogs in one very large, well-funded machine.

Let's use a random example. Someone comes into the emergency room:

1. They're going to be seen by the administrative staff, the front desk person. Then from there, they're going to be wheeled back to a room where they will wait and continuously gather information through various monitors.

   The first thing they're going to be asked for is an insurance card. If you ever have been in a hospital, you know that's the first thing you're asked for, almost like they run to the door asking for it. If you don't have an insurance card, they start getting upset with you and start grilling you line-by-line – they're trained to know that patients with no insurance aren't a money fountain and are practically 'no good' to the corporation.

   Feel like you're on a conveyor belt yet?

2. At some point, a health team member will enter the room and gather some more history like a health rundown, physical, and a few other factors. These are called 'DRG codes' and can only be done by a trained medical professional in person.

DRG codes are the turning point for the hospital, as a medical team member has had to perform an assessment. The initial bill will be based on that DRG code. Patients don't realize that most physicians are told to bill out higher DRG codes so that the hospital can get reimbursed for the highest cost possible.

Let's say that this patient has pneumonia or congestive heart failure – easy to say, as these two are the most common diagnoses in the US. That's an automatic entry ticket into a hospital. Dollar signs!

3. From here, the patient goes through the system. Every test that's ordered on them, every tiny thing is done on that little barcode on their wrist. Using that barcode is a charge being applied.

If you ever look at your bill in detail, you'll notice a ton of 'suspicious but legal' charges.

A single pill of aspirin should not cost 12 dollars to administer. A bag of saltwater in an IV shouldn't cost 100 dollars, either. It cost the medical supply company, at most, a dollar to make.

All of these charges are totally legal and backed up by insurance companies and the government, which, remember, help to fund these large health corporations through the contributions of grants, federal aid money, and tax breaks. Any time laws that could potentially change up the system are quickly shot down, remember that both the insurance and health systems have highly-paid lobbyists just waiting to squash any part of said reforms. Remember how much these systems make each day –

they can easily afford this legal bribery – and won't be feeling a crunch anytime soon.

Ripped Off

Time for a little math.

For a doctor such as myself, my direct pay cut of a cardiologic procedure is anywhere from $500 to $1,000, depending on the case's complexity. Sounds pretty good, right? That means anywhere from around $4,000 - $8,000 a day!

Well, factor in that for the same procedure, a procedure where my hands were doing the work, the hospital would bring in around $120,000. On a busy day, I could make them close to a million dollars in revenue.

One day, looking at my pay stubs and knowing what was going on, my brain started to spin.

"What are they doing differently? Those executives need me to perform the procedures, but it seems like I'm being shortchanged. If I don't do a procedure, they don't make a dime."

This is where the business part of my mind started kicking in, there in the middle of the hospital of the very system that was seemingly taking advantage of my skills.

"I need to work smarter, not harder. I need to find my freedom. I'm done running on the hamster wheel."

Outpatient

The outpatient cath lab was born.

Imagine your routine neighborhood freestanding surgery center – cruise over to your closest health park, and there will be a few of them. Aesthetic Plastic Surgery centers are the most common of these setups. These doctor-run clinics are freestanding aspects of the hospital system that aren't directly owned or related to them; instead, they work in a congenial fashion with large area hospitals. Of course, these doctors, including myself, are taking on many more risks personally, business-wise, and professionally, but the financial and professional rewards are extraordinary, compared to giving a large cut to a hospital system.

That's the entire 'shadow economy' in a nutshell. A process that isn't really taught – one under our noses but generally misunderstood, and much less taught.

On my clinic's opening day, I unlocked the doors and stepped in, perhaps a little tentatively, but continued telling myself inside – "I can do this." I had to do it myself, but I had to do it for my patients and staff as well – the medical business is one of extreme accountability. Any corner you turn, you'll run into someone who is relying on you. That is a heavy burden, but also one that constantly reminds you of how important you are.

OUTCOMES

This is the same concept as knowing the value of Google or Tesla stock years before the companies were even founded – we all look at our decisions and pound ourselves over the head with mallets, knowing we should have invested when we had the chance.

Prices for these companies have risen each year. Five, ten, fifteen…Pound! Pound! Pound!

Branching Out

Hindsight is 20/20; that's why I believe it is important for every person, from patient to doctor, to know the system they're feeding into every time they go into a hospital. Don't get me wrong, hospitals save lives every day, but at what cost?

I'm at the stage of shouting with a megaphone – Future doctors of America – know this! Get out of the hamster wheel! You can help your patients and yourselves much more efficiently on your own! When you are charged up, your services reflect that fact – a tired, unhappy doctor is vastly less effective than one that is well-rested!

Living at Work

Laws are changing, and we have to be aware of them. It is either that or be caught unaware when it is too late.

When I was doing my residency, I did anywhere from 100 to 120 hours a week of training. That means practically living in the hospital – those stories you've heard of residents simply crashing in an empty patient room are true – and paired with this sleeplessness and brain strain, you see a lot of patients, and when you see a lot of patients, you see a lot of catastrophes.

The worst-case scenario in the healthcare field and many others happens when you come into a situation that catches you off-guard and you panic. That strange, hard-to-treat case comes in on a stretcher, and their life has to be saved. You aren't sure what to do. The adrenaline kicks in. Combine that with being tired, and you've got a ticking time-bomb waiting to go off.

We've seen it happen, and we're told about it in medical school. A doctor sees something new and strange, and they panic. They literally freeze in the middle of surgery, their patient fading, and they 'fold their hands,' not knowing what to do. This situation is the same as any other time in life. However, again, just like in life, if you've seen a situation before, you're less likely to panic, no matter what the circumstances may be.

Let's add this up. Let's say the training is seven years, then add

30-40 hours each week. Over six years that's 1500 – 2000 hours. That's a whole lot of time to see things.

Help Yourself

Within the past few years, *The New York Times* evaluated individuals who went to medical school and became doctors.

That's comparing someone in their early thirties, the doctor, to someone in their mid-forties, the MBA-holder. It's easy to see that the MBA-holder has probably brought in much more cash than the young doctor in question. The doctor is carrying debt, has been in school for 10 years, residency training is busy building a new practice, and lumping on more debt – great! Oh, right, and add on a family if that applies!

However, if you're looking at the long term, the doctor will catch up and overtake those with an MBA. How? By opening their own clinics. That's a combination of the MBA holder's business skills, with a layer of medical experience over the top.

For example, if you have an office, you've got staff – how many staff do you really need to function? How much office square footage do you need to pay rent on?

If you start really maximizing, rather than overloading and overspending, you'll save enough money where you cut that gap down versus those with an MBA, then eclipse them and forge ahead.

Debt Factor

As far as debt is concerned, it is the largest, scariest hurdle out there for anyone.

Let's face it – we're doctors, not accountants. Most of us don't know anything about interest rates, how to offset our loans, and how to get lines of credit. It is true that most doctors even struggle to get a mortgage or car loan the moment they walk into any bank out there. The person who is a business to everyone else is a victim.

The moment this will change for doctors is the moment we all accept that we're dollar signs on a chart for hospitals and insurance systems. It is time that we acknowledge and understand this fact, then use it to our advantage. We're a business. Time to act like it! Do you see business owners struggling to get homes or cars due to their business-related debt? Of course not, the law protects them. We can do this too!

R&R

Part of the reason that we flounder, even under normal circumstances, is that we strain our minds.

Ask any doctor out there, including me, if we can generally regard the human brain as a type of 'muscle,' and like any muscle in the body, repeated, relentless use will cause the muscle to be strained and eventually break down or enter a period of forced recovery.

To allow our minds to recover, we must rest and relax – hands down, bar none. Otherwise, at some point, that muscle reaction will kick in and turn us into shuffling 'zombies,' learning nothing, feeling little, and simply dealing with life as it comes. That's no way to learn, work, or live! At this point, taking some time to rest and relax is purely humanitarian!

It may be 15 to 30 minutes a day of just reading something you want – to challenge yourself with something new. It could be to learn something totally out of your league, or hey, even to learn more information about your prospective field. Hey! Imagine if I never read up on cardiology – I just might have a line of patients out the door who are angry that they aren't receiving the most up-to-date standards of care!

MAKING THE PROFESSION WORK FOR US

I remember putting a talk together for career day with my son when he was in middle school.

Of course, all of the kids wanted to hear about grizzly operating room stories or the time I jumped into an ambulance and helped to save a life. Remember, middle schoolers generally only have television shows and movies as a frame of reference – they have the joy of 'not knowing any better.'

The kids were shocked when I didn't quite go into that but explained the business side of health.

I spoke about the office building that a doctor uses. They should own it. That's not all, though; they need to follow through with a lease-back. The doctor leases the property back to himself via two different corporations to risk avert and maximize deductions.

Talk about a room of dumbfounded kids. Their definition of a doctor went from 'that guy at the hospital who fixes people up' to a 'real business doctor who fixes people up.'

Now that we're done chuckling about me shocking a room full of middle-schoolers, let's do some thinking.

Imagine a doctor owns his building. No payments to a landlord, that's somewhere from \$3,000-\$5,000 per month. You're saving anywhere from \$30,000-\$50,000 a year. That's a whole lot of procedures.

Imagine having 10 to 15 to 20 offices. Now that's how to monetize yourself as a business! A doctor who does real estate – real estate for his own healthcare business – taking care of patients and himself. These savings give the doctor more space for free time to learn, relax, and be a productive member of society – the service quality is better through the doctor not living and working in the office all day and all night.

All I can say is that I wish someone would've taught me this from the beginning. Well, I suppose I've driven home the point for this book, haven't I?

CHAPTER 2

FROM COLLEGE TO THE HOSPITAL

It is a long, tumultuous process for students.

What you don't know, you don't know. This foresight is important in medicine. You'll either need to know what you don't know at the moment or find a quick way to find out what you need to know to save a life.

We're taught this in medical school – basically, how to be effective. How to anticipate worst-case scenarios.

How do we get there?

1. Get good grades in high school; that's the basic starting point.
2. From there, you've then got the concept of four years of college, and, of course, it is always better to attend a high-prestige university. A medical school is going to jump at an ivy league name over a commuter school in the middle of nowhere. You spend four years there, get good grades, do a lot of extracurriculars, and hope to walk across the stage with honors.
3. Now it's time to really take the deep dive from college to medical school, which just might be one of the most difficult

transitions in your life. You're going to have to take the MCAT exam. MCAT, the Medical College Admissions Test, is the most difficult exam I've taken in my life, I can say for sure.

Note:

The MCAT is not like the SAT, which everyone knows and talks about. The MCAT is there to specifically weed out the elite from the non-elite. It is the great leveler that shows medical schools which students can really make it through.

MEDICAL SCHOOL LIFE IS TOUGH

Let's start out with the hard facts of the matter. You don't know what you don't know – but the good news is that it's all okay.

If you don't know the answer, you will be a hundred percent wrong, and it's going to affect someone's life. In fact, a wrong medical diagnosis could kill someone outright or sentence them to a long, painful process of suffering from their illness.

Let's propose that you get into medical school; it's a lower number of admissions there, obviously. Four more years of extremely intense studying and scrutiny. From there, you must apply for your residency.

Long Days Ahead

Finding a residency is kind of like a draft process that you see in football, baseball, or basketball, where new doctors are picked by priority into a training program, taking into account their GPA, honors, and other factors. Of course, the top member of the class will get placed first, then the second, third, and on down the tree all the way to the bottom.

In my case, my residency was for three years of internal medicine studies in a hospital system in Michigan with Michigan State University. Internal medicine is a primary level of training and residency – if you're looking to enter into a specialty, the climb gets that much harder.

Got through that stage? Great. The next step, in my example, is Cardiology. That was another three years. From there, I went into another specialty called Interventional Cardiology; in that stage, there were maybe a hundred graduates a year at the most.

Needless to say, the competition gets nastily aggressive the higher you go. For just a rough comparison, there are 1,300,000 lawyers compared to 3255 Interventional cardiologists. The NFL has 1695 active NFL players. This gives you an idea of how competitive and difficult it is. Not to mention the fact that the expectations continue to rise. Think that all of this sounds incredibly intense?

Do you want a heart surgeon who can't map out the quadrants of the heart? I sure wouldn't.

TO THE ROOKIES

There's a certain aspect that you have to live up to as a doctor in training. You are your own business. You are a walking piece of business, and you need to understand the concept of how to monetize yourself, as those hospital systems that are bound to come calling after graduation day aren't interested in your personal wealth; they are interested in pulling you in to act as the scalpel in their hand to extract money from patient's wallets.

Be who you are and do it in a maximum way.

Running the Final Leg

What's with all of this? Why do it?

We are treated like this, almost like going through a mental meat grinder, in order to prepare us for any possible situation in one of the millions of possibilities that could walk through the door. No matter how horrible the situation, a doctor can never be allowed to freeze up. The moment you freeze is the moment that mistakes are made.

As the old saying goes, 'don't hate the player, hate the game.' Really, if you think about it, it is the same concept in life, to the transition to a work environment or business from the fun-filled years of being in college. Our professors have already seen what we're going to experience. They know what is going to go on out there.

We love to watch medical shows, read medical books, and act out our doctor dreams in video games, but the professors in schools know what's actually happening out there and the true consequences. The writer doesn't just write another book, the actor doesn't just stand up from the table, and we aren't able to close out of the game. People really do die.

FROM A PATIENT'S EYES

Next time you're sitting in that waiting room, you may want to rethink your opinions when you're waiting in that room, seemingly for hours and hours.

'Waiting room' is really a different name for the process that means the patients come to see 'Dr. Right.' You know, doctors are learning as you're learning because everything is not in a textbook.

Medicine is changing dramatically. You can see based on what's happening in reality. It isn't like it used to be 20 years ago, where everything's on Google being at your fingertips to search. So, as a result, the doctor can't tell you one doctor that thinks he knows more about COVID than another doctor because if they do, that's not true, and they'll easily be caught in their own lie. Just as much as the lay public knows, everybody else knows.

In return, I would lower your expectations when you're going to ask your doctor about conditions. His answer is going to be informed by two things – his experience and his reading.

After that, he's going to tell you, based on the experience that he's had over the last 10, 20 years or whatever time period it may be, that he's got 'X' opinion. He's got to combine those two action items and then present them to you as his education deduction. We're not here in a dictatorship where we tell you what to do as a patient. We offer our opinions and leave you to decide.

It is important for patients to understand that a medical student doesn't know what an attending doctor of twenty years knows, and an attending doctor of twenty years knows much more than, say, a doctor of five. Every year, everyone gains a little more experience.

I tell you to be open-minded and unemotional when it comes to making decisions and enjoy what you do well. If the passion is gone, your ability to develop skills will fly the coop.

RESIDENCY – THE REAL WORLD

The first year out of medical school, you're going to have an attending physician looking over your shoulder to make sure you don't, for lack of better words, kill someone with your lack of experience.

Let's look at it as if we were cutting up a block of Swiss cheese. Don't worry, stay with me. Close your eyes, think, and picture that block of cheese until the image is clear in your mind. Pale yellow and full of holes. You've got a scalpel in your hand. Start taking off slices lengthwise, horizontally, and lay them out. Got it? Great!

Now, take those slices and begin piling them back on top of each other, as if you were going to 'rebuild' that block of cheese. No matter what, you can never reconnect those pieces, right? Even so, you probably won't be able to match the holes back together to perfectly combine as the whole block, as it was before.

It's not too uncommon in the medical world to meet patients who are a lot like that block of Swiss cheese. They've been through so many doctors, treatments, and processes that it seems like they'll never be whole again. The only time those holes matchup is when a patient passes away and becomes one with the Earth again.

Suffice it to say, when these patients come to you, you're about to make a few more slices on their cheese block. Scary stuff, right? It is scary.

Knowing Your Place

Usually, the 'super-specialist,' such as a surgeon, internal medicine specialist, or disease expert, has the most responsibility with their respective client's case. They are constantly the last line of defense.

When an internal medicine, family practice doctor, or pediatrician puts in for a consultation, they are getting a recommendation from a specialist – let's say that the example is a consultation with a cardiologist. The referring doctor has spotted an issue and can't handle it on their own, so they pass the patient up the ladder to the next level of expertise for information. The patient will continue to climb up the ladder until they receive the treatment or information they need to handle their case. Sometimes, in complicated cases, four, five, and six doctors could be involved from different areas of knowledge.

As you can see, the answer is never "I don't know" but always "we know who to go to in order to find out."

Let's say you're a medicine specialist, the 'super-specialist.' You're the last line of defense – after that, there's nobody else. The patient has climbed up as far as they can, and it is a long fall back down. It is a huge emotional burden.

Is that emotional burden something that you can handle? The stakes are real.

Learn from Experience, But Take a Breath

Everybody says you learn from experience, and you learn from your mistakes. This is a field where you don't want to learn from your mistakes because that one mistake that you make could cost someone's life. It could cost your license. Hundreds of thousands of dollars and your chosen career down the drain.

The keynote here is to continue educating yourself. You're going to need to read more about:

- Disease processes.
- New treatments.
- How to refer patients out to the right doctor.

Read and study enough about that situation you want to avoid. Be ready to become prepared for any challenge or situation.

Read, read, read. You've got to read an extra 15 to 30 minutes a day of something that's unrelated to anything you're doing. Your mind is a muscle; it does eventually need to switch gears and relax, or you, as a doctor in training, or someone interested in medicine knows, it will snap and strain itself.

KNOW YOUR DOLLAR SIGNS

Again, the hospital system sees you as a walking dollar sign. Somewhere, on some spreadsheet in the accounting and HR departments, you are a badge number with a revenue-generating amount attached to your name.

The question is, though, what do you see yourself as? Do you see yourself as a blip on a corporate monetization chart? The healthy answer is a resounding "no," and for most medical students, I would say over 98% don't see themselves that way.

It doesn't stop in the walls of the hospital, though. Keep in mind: you have a name, but you are a number when you call the pharmacy. They ask you for what's called an NPI number. That's your National Practitioner Identifier. A unique number is assigned as your ID so that pharmacies are able to know who is calling.

In the end, you have to look at yourself as a widget in every situation. It gets more complicated from across the desk. You have to look at that person across the desk and understand that the person you're looking at is a widget, and they're learning as you're learning. The system looks at them as dollar signs as well, a walking blank check issued by an insurance company.

In Debt

Even in this case, patients actually see you as a dollar sign because they think, 'Oh, this doctor is making so much money that he's going to charge me then head out to his Ferrari and drive to his lake house.' They don't realize or even think of the amount of debt you have. You've paid hundreds of thousands of dollars for college, hundreds of thousands of dollars to medical school. You're likely in more debt than they are.

The moment you clock out, you're starting a family, and you're young – now you've got kids, a mortgage, car payments, and probably some credit card bills.

You've got this psychological concept of I've-got-to-live-the-lifestyle. "I'm a doctor. I need a big house. I need a fancy car." You are falling into the same trap that your patients have fallen into, …the hamster wheel.

Avoid that pitfall.

Do you want that fancy car? It is a constantly depreciating asset. The car is not going to appreciate like a house – skip the car, buy a house, something that you can sell later for more than you paid initially. In the grand scheme of things, you've already done this, going to medical school.

Everyone needs to educate themselves with 15 minutes of reading on what a mortgage is, how much interest you pay in the first 10 years of it, versus the last 15 years you pay on a 25-year mortgage or a 30-year mortgage. There are savings to be found and money to be made, no matter what the original purchase price of the home is.

As a doctor, you're smart enough to know the difference. There's no excuse. Then again, there's no excuse for the general public, either.

I'm going to tell you, avoid the lifestyle because the name of that lifestyle is "debt."

LOOKING BACK – GOOD FOR ME, GOOD FOR YOU

Okay, you've gotten through residency, and now you are an attending physician yourself. You know what you have become. There's no going back. The responsibility is on you.
You have become something.

When you're a resident and graduating from interventional cardiology, in my case, you don't know what's going on outside. You're in this small world. You're in this small 'little' niche – where the outside world doesn't bother you until it enters through the door, struggling to survive, out of the blue.

Meanwhile, during all of this, you're with a bunch of other alphas, all on different levels, and all fighting for the same pool of resources on one end of the spectrum, and on the other end, selfishly, they want to prove themselves better than you.

It gets more intense though, since, sure, there's a God complex involved, because you're saving people from dying from heart attacks, cancer, and every disease under the sun. You don't see that at first, but then you begin seeing it in little streaks.

From there, you see the massive power of these large, complicated medical groups. It's all about money to them at the start, and it's about money in the end. They will do anything to get at it.

An 'X' On Your Heart

Should you go out into the market on your own, the hospital system and physician groups will attempt to push you out. You're not protected. If there is a mistake, the hospital will come after you. If you do something wrong, the private group will come after you because they see you as competition. They'd rather see you go down in flames than succeed.

You're in this world alone. Scary and lonely are the operative words.

You are in the Serengeti. You are on a safari, you are all alone in those thousands of square miles, and you are the prey. You're not a predator; even though you think you're a predator at that time, you won't become a predator until you've been attacked and survived at least once – and you know it's coming.

Know the Unpredictability of the Beast

As an example, during my interventional cardiology training at the University of Utah, a patient came into the emergency room having a heart attack. An active, potentially lethal heart attack.

Normally, when you're training, you want to do everything, and why not? Your attending physician is there to supervise everything you do and step in if need be. On this afternoon, he simply looked at me and said, "Take the case."

As I'm scrubbing up to start, another active case stumbled in through the door. Another active heart attack. He's ushered into another room, leaving me minutes to work on the first case, then move on to him.

My attending doctor comes back and starts scrubbing up as well – he'll take over the first case, mine, and I'll take the second. In response, I walk over to his sink after he is sterile and contaminate him. His response, "F@*! you contaminated me."

I purposefully contaminated him. He'd have to leave, scrub up again, then come back. I had bought myself ten minutes to do both cases.

In short, since I can't break HIPPA rules, the patient did great. Once it was all over and I could take a few seconds to break away, the attending doctor found me, and in the back of my mind, I was expecting a beat down.

"You did great." he said, "and I know what you did."

Around eight months afterward, that same exact scenario happens again. He's not there this time. I am in the real world with no backup help. It's just me.

Obviously, I'm cocky when I'm in training because I do have somebody to back me up if things go wrong. Someone to clean up any mess. He's there to go to that second case if it comes in that quickly, but this time, he's not there. I'm alone.

I have to finish that first case. I don't know what I'm expecting. I don't know what's going to happen. The guy may crash, meaning he's getting close to death, and there may be complications, and then I'm stuck. Meanwhile, during all this, the other guy is still waiting. He may die. You may have both patients die. What's going to happen?

You don't know. We can't predict the future.

You've got training, you know how to do it, but there's also this element of surprise that comes into play. Do you know training versus reality? How do you prepare yourself for this? Can you prepare yourself for this?

Facing the Facts

You know, I hate to say this, but new graduates don't have as much training.

In fact, I remember doing 100 to 120 hours a week when I could get them in. Now they do 60-80 hours a week and cap it at that, generally. If you add 40 hours a week extra for that extra year of training, that's thousands of hours of training they've missed. That's thousands of hours that another doctor did not get, that I did. I was lucky, though my obligations weren't as strict, and I could do that.

If you're unable to get that experience, you need to read and be prepared for what's going to happen in future situations. It may not be hands-on time, but it is as good as you can get, given your circumstances.

ABL – Always Be Learning

During all this time, you're learning about the pitfalls. You're learning about the complications that could happen in a heart attack patient. You're learning about how to manage time and prepare yourself...

Personally, you know that those extra five minutes are going to affect someone's life. I love doing surgery and procedures. I love being an interventional cardiologist. I enjoy it, but I've met plenty of doctors who do not enjoy what they do, know exactly why they don't love it, and they don't care about learning anymore. They're just there to get paid to get rid of their debt. They're miserable. They're not happy.

Don't be this kind of professional—in medicine especially.

Are You Happy?

Whatever job you have, you need to be happy with that job. I don't care what it is that you do, whether it's someone that works in sanitation on the side of the road, someone that loves to climb mountains as a tour guide, or a nurse in a hospital.

Don't chase after the money – the money is an illusion thought up by Hollywood to create great doctor characters that make us want to binge-watch television shows. When you chase money, the money runs. You need to chase what you are happy with and enjoy doing, and when you're doing that, you're going to be successful, regardless of what it is.

Chase after the idea of saving lives and making a difference.

CHAPTER 3

BUSINESS 101

When you come out of residency and training, ready to go into the world of medicine, you're set forth into a world of freedom, school debt, and boundless opportunity. There are a lot of ways to go right and a lot of ways to go wrong. Unfortunately, the warning signs for either whizz by at such a quick pace that you won't have time to read them.

YOU'RE IN BUSINESS

No matter if you're running a restaurant, a candy store, a dentist's office, or a makeup counter, many aspects of business are the same, despite the ongoing notion within the public that they are all run differently, when really, all the basics are the same.

The true difference is that we have different rules to the restaurant businesses. They have their health codes, and we have our HIPAA rules. Break a health code, and you could get slapped with a heavy fine. Break a HIPAA role, and you could lose your medical license.

That's a big difference.

No Protection

Unfortunately, that difference scares many medical students away from opening their own clinic or business. Like we've explored, that independence means there are no high-paid lawyers and coverage that large medical systems offer if something goes wrong. Going your own way means exactly that – to leave the herd.

Bills

There's payroll, rent, insurance, utilities – and those are just the basics to open the doors. There's an endless list of possibilities after that – maybe a coffee bar in the lobby for patients, professional memberships, advertising?

To make things easier, let's break down the top expenses:

1. **Salaries and payroll?** This item is the single-handedly most expensive line item in any office. Alongside the point of having to pay them out, are there ways to cheapen the blow without degrading service? For example, if you've got multiple offices and they only run half a day a week for a total of two days per week, staff can bounce between locations, rather than having a staff for each office. You could potentially quarter or halve the bill just with that decision alone!

2. **Rent or mortgage?** Ideally, you'll want to own your own building, of course. Need to knock out a wall to expand a treatment room? No calling the landlord, begging for permission, and signing piles of forms! In terms of owning your own facility, you're paying into your own rent as both landlord and tenant. Unfortunately, as a starting doctor, if you can't do that financially in the beginning, then you've got to find somewhere that it's economically feasible.

3. **What's your mix?** Most don't see it exactly as an overhead expense, but it's the demographics – what types of patients are you going to be seeing in your area. Will the problems you're treating and cases you will be seeing pay the bills?

4. **Got medical supplies?** For the same reasons that people love Costco, buying in bulk means a cheaper bottom line. This is especially great for doctors who control multiple offices, as bulk orders can be split up between offices, meaning less wastage.
5. **Got the drive?** Is your essence, drive, passion, and expertise going to drive the office(s) you own to excel and progress?

FINDING YOUR BALANCE

In founding a medical office, let alone any business, the true work is in finding the balance of operations paired with budgets. As a business owner, you must face down the barrel of growing responsibly in a market that could flip on a dime.

The First Days

In the beginning, you're not seeing enough patients, and you're not busy enough. This will always be the case. Remember, you're a fresh face up against the hospital and group system – there will be bigger fish out there able to pull in clients much faster in every form – public reviews, referrals, word of mouth.

Payroll Woes

Your payroll, in this case, will be higher because you've got to have staff on hand that aren't fully busy during the day but are necessary to keep on hand in order to perform your line of business. This is one of a few times in business where the old tough love line of "suck it up" applies.

Traffic Flow

We aren't talking about your parking lot! – Well, not explicitly, at least.

As your clinic builds up, for example, you've got 10 patients coming in through the day. That's well and good; however, you've got to build that up to 15 patients, then 20 patients a day, then 25 patients a day; and then your staff size has to increase once you're bursting at the seams to meet the demands of traffic coming through the door. When that time comes, can your clinic afford to add new staff? If so, you're on the right path; if not, it may be time to evaluate and cut back.

The only way to truly perform traffic management well is to always be on top of changes that are coming up – always know when a new staff member needs to be hired, or a new room needs to be added. Traffic flow is all about making changes before things have an opportunity to get backed up.

Is your quality of care staying at the same level or growing? That's the ultimate goal.

The Marketing Baton

From here, you have two choices –

1. Start spending a marketing budget.
2. Bring in enough patients for word-of-mouth marketing that you become a known presence in your community.

The idea of saying "Hi, I'm Doctor X, doctor extraordinaire, step this way!" to an endless line of ready-to-play clients from day one – it doesn't work that way.

You're here, just like any other business, be it a restaurant or an Instagram influencer, for lack of better words, to market and get your name out there using whatever method you can. This can work in both positive and negative ways.

'Good' and 'Bad' Doctors

When you spend time with a patient, 90% of the time before you walk into the room, you've already reviewed their chart – you know what's going on with them, your likely suggestions, tests you're going to pursue, questions you're going to ask. Your patient's chart is essentially an extension of their voice – they speak to you through it.

You've already made up your mind and decision before even seeing them.

By the time you enter the consultation room, you've already completed a percentage of the case. Your face time with the patient will be spent building a relationship and gathering any little bits of unknown information that could be helpful in confirming your decision.

If you're seeing 20, 30, 40 patients for the day, you've got a short amount of time, and you start pushing yourself to go to the next patient who is already waiting in a nearby consultation room. Is there truly time to think over your decisions and be sure that you're correct?

That's where you do two things in the consultation time with your patient:

1. You're going to get the most pertinent information related to their health history.
2. You're going to get the most pertinent information related to their personal history because this is where you build that bond and build that business relationship with the patient in question. This, for the lack of better wording, is the building up for the "sales" transaction.

"How's your granddaughter doing in college?"

"You mentioned your son being in a school play. How'd he do?"

In this moment, you're building the ladder up to the sweet spot between quantity, quality, and care. The moment you reach it, like a button on the wall, you hit it as many times as you can before it moves on. The higher the "score" you get, the more likely the patient is to come back.

This is the difference between a 'good' doctor and, and for lack of a better word, a 'bad' doctor in the court of professional and public opinion.

When you go into surgery, and an unforeseen circumstance arises, a good surgeon is able to come out of that outcome without worrying one bit about it and save the patient's life.

The bad doctor, on the other hand, will not be able to perform and, for lack of a better description, panics in the moment, leading to them forgetting what they need to know – and this can be deadly in the worst of cases, and in the best of these cases, end in a botched surgery.

You want to be known for your best outcomes; you want to be known as "the surgeon that saves lives."

It boils down to a simple philosophy:

When someone puts their life in your hands, you have to be sure that you'll be able to pull them through – if you aren't sure, you shouldn't do that surgery.

You want to be known as the best in the business. This policy will take you there.

It's Business 101, simple as that.

Understanding the 'Back-End'

Never underestimate the value of an administrator – I can speak on this topic from my own adventures in business.

When first starting my own clinic, I had three office members at the front desk keeping our operation afloat, with a few nurses helping in the back. This usually went fine, until some days when we were running 40-50 patients seemingly back-to-back-to-back, leaving me feeling stressed and spread thin.

On this day in question, we're behind by over an hour. Patients are getting upset, asking to reschedule, and further clogging up the works. One of the office staff came to the back to ask me a question about the codes for a patient who just left – feeling the pressure, I snapped at her.

She starts crying. At that moment, the office changed.

I could hear my own voice running through my mind. "I can't do this. I need an administrator to run the front of the house. I'm going to hurt people at this rate. I'm going to have upset patients. I need help."

That led to me hiring an administrator, a full-time administrator – that person oversaw the multiple offices that we were in, the HR department in terms of bringing on new staff, ran the billing department, and slowly started transitioning into the other smaller aspects that our offices needed.

Many studies have been done which show that we, as human beings, aren't great at multitasking. Our brains can, to some degree, but we aren't meant for carrying out multiple tasks at once. With each additional task on the load, performance drops. Your administration team is good at administration. You need to do what you've been trained for – medicine.

I've talked to a lot of physicians throughout my time in the medical business. Most of them are horrible businesspeople but great physicians, and that's fine. However, when you do business well, when you have 'business genes', it's very difficult for you to give up that side. For me, that was the most difficult thing: letting someone else run the business of the clinic while I used my training in medicine. The clinic is my baby that I've built from scratch, and now I'm letting someone else take care of my baby. It feels strange and putting the trust and faith into them to run the business side of things feels even more foreign.

Don't get me wrong, though. At the same time, I still had my foot in the door as the chief officer – only a chief officer with split responsibilities. Small, mundane activities go away. Only a few large issues each week. Never forget that you're a business owner at the end of the day.

Managing Your Personal Brand

Great! You've put in all the work necessary to get your clinic open, but what's there to do now? Well, there's the obvious – bringing in patients.

Ten years ago, this conversation would be much simpler. We'd be talking about newspaper ads, billboards, all of the traditional methods of marketing. Now, these options are still out there, but there's a new major player in the marketing business that just steamrolls all other options out there – Facebook, Instagram, Google... the big names we all know.

Websites, Social Media, Your Patients, and You

Think of your business(es) as a tree. The trunk is your main practice, seeing and treating clients. However, with any healthy tree, there are plenty of branches that catch rays of sun and drops of rain to keep that tree trunk healthy.

That sun and rain, in our case, is made up of referrals and clients coming through the doors. Maybe they connected with something on your website's blog and wanted to finally have a concern checked out, maybe you successfully treated a friend or family member of theirs, maybe they saw you in a newspaper article – whatever the source may be, they will find their way to you.

The canopy, the collection of all of your leaves, creates your presence.

Put Stock in Yourself

In my own case, I built a book of clients through venues big and small. For example, back in the beginning, and even now, it wasn't uncommon to find me at big RV parks, senior centers, golf tournaments, and more – up on the stage, speaking about heart health. After those talks, I'd have potential clients and referrals lined up, ready to speak with me privately for a few minutes.

Know Your Patient-Base

Suffice it to say, I've always known who to market to. Being an Interventional Cardiologist, I know I'm dealing with an elderly population, sufferers of heart conditions from a lifetime of American lifestyles and diets.

Be Memorable

That's the rule of the game under this category.

Yes, I'm a heart doctor who went out and got a 1-800-HEART phone number. It sounds tacky, but it worked. Patients are customers at the end of the day, and catchy marketing will always catch the mind and heart of a customer before any other format, just behind word of mouth and personal recommendations.

Craft Your Website

Make it obvious what you want patients to do when they come to your practice's website. Would you like them to sign up for your newsletter? Do you want to set up a free consultation with them? Do you want them to make an appointment with you? Make sure you understand your message and how you want patients to react.

Do you offer online bookings for initial consultations? It isn't a bad idea. Your medical practice's website is accessible 24 hours a day, seven days a week, which means it can continue to attract new patients even after office hours. Make it easy for patients to arrange an appointment and sign up for your services by allowing them to do so online.

Word of Mouth is Still King

I had had an individual in the hospital having a heart attack – totally like on a TV show – the man is half-clothed on a gurney, blasted through the doors, into the operating room, with me chasing from behind. As I'm running alongside, the man looks up at me.

"You're doing this? You're too young."

I've heard it all, it feels like, so I ignored it for a moment. We all say things when we're in a panic.

"You're younger than my son. How can you do this?"

My response was "It's either me, or you die." I simply tell him, unsure of what else to tell him than the truth. I am pretty forward when I speak with my patients.

The man takes a breath.

"Go ahead."

The surgery went through just fine, and afterward, I learned a little about the man. He was some kind of big wig, you know, a few thousand employees under his belt and a few hundred million in his bank account. With the way I spoke to him, it wasn't that he just accepted my age; he accepted my confidence.

As a result, that led to him marketing my clinic more, sending more patients to me, and then their insurance company started helping us. As a result, the firefighters, the local police, they all started getting more involved in our practice – all because I was confident and saved the man's life.

Hold Up! Did You Get Clearance?

When you have a patient, and you're going to publicize them on social media, you must get a disclaimer. HIPAA is a killer.

1. **You must get an NDA** (Non-Disclosure Agreement). Bar none. No chances to take. No dice to roll. If there's no signature, there's no green light. Work with a lawyer to create an NDA that clearly states their story or image can be used, but not together.
2. **Never use real names**. It's very difficult to use a patient's real name, again, HIPAA. Sharing a photo and medical information about the person is highly illegal. Take a look at medicine advertisements where 'real users' are shown. There generally will be some subtext that 'paid actors' are being used. This is the usual way big pharmaceutical and hospital groups get around the rule – use edited testimonials paired with fake names and the photos of actors. This 'abstraction' of the patient and their story is legal.

Patients will understand what you're doing, and if the NDA is signed, they can't return later, saying you never had permission to share their story or image.

Example: Plastic and Dental Surgery
The most common example of this in practice is within the plastic and dental surgery community – clients are often asked if photos of their before and after can be shared. The NDA to do so is often collected in the first batch of paperwork signed before even a consultation is carried out. Think back to the last time you were at the dentist or orthodontist, if you've never had plastic surgery – you've likely seen examples of corrected smiles hanging on the walls in the waiting room. Yet another example!

When the patient comes back to meet with you, you'll have a note on their chart saying whether they'll participate in taking photos or not. Easy!

THE MEDICINE BUSINESS

In medical school, we're taught anatomy, physiology, and about the ins and outs of the human body – there's never a class on business. That part is saved until you interact with insurance or Medicaid yourself in an attempt to get paid.

In this example, you're treating a patient, great! Now they've left, and you need to take care of billing. You're unable to do your job without having a billing code, also known as a 'DRG Code.'

You dig around, getting the information you need, and finally, find the proper billing code. From here, you've got to use the proper form to send into their insurance provider – this is the way you're paid, after all!

In this case, you're in luck – the patient is using Medicare and not private insurance. There's a simple form that's followed for Medicare, and it all can be done digitally. You start filling in the blanks down the page until you reach the 'send' button.

It really is that simple, and we aren't taught it.

We've got this whole protocol:

1. Get their current history.
2. Get their past medical history.
3. Get their allergies.
4. Get their medications.
5. Get their review systems.

It's a process. This protocol is almost like a hamster wheel.

We're not taught these other items; it's almost like you're looking on the internet for what to do. "How do I properly bill a patient as a doctor?" In school, we're taught everything just up to the cusp of the business aspect. No wonder joining a hospital system is so attractive, right? You can have a whole department do this for you!

In all reality, these are things that should be done in 15 to 30 minutes. Talk about the hospital system taking advantage of gaps in knowledge for their own gain!

Billing Codes

You've reviewed your patient's chart, spent time with them, diagnosed them, reviewed their history. It seems like your part of the job is nearly over. The problem is, though, the patient needs a few layers of care – that means complications in two realms, the medical side, which you have a handle on, and the billing side.

The first step is to figure out diagnosis codes to enter – these codes tell the insurance company exactly what is going on, like their own form of shorthand.

When Should I Get It Done?

You have options!

1. There are physicians who like to do the billing right then and there after seeing the patient because it's easier, as they don't forget.
   The downside is that, of course, that eats up time in seeing new patients if it is a busy day.
2. From here, there are physicians who like to do this at the end of the day – going through it all, reviewing through all their charts for every patient, and entering each code.

Of course, the downside here is that this will eat up time at the end of the day, taking an extra hour or two, and depending on how tired you are, may introduce mistakes. Besides, you have plenty to do after you clock off anyway, right?

Building Your System

Building out your system is more important than the actual concept of picking the correct DRG codes, as strange as it sounds.

The system of sitting down and reviewing the patient's chart prior, then reviewing again when you walk in and start the consultation is different, because then you can anticipate what your codes are going to be and what your level of care is going to be after leaving the room.

The homework doesn't end just because the patient is out of the room – in fact, this step is just as important as this is your paycheck at the end of the day.

Go Third-Party?

My own clinic operates using a third-party billing company – and quite frankly, I suggest it for everyone.

You've got two choices:

- Bring in a third-party billing company to code your bills for you.
- Have an in-house biller who you pay a salary to undertake all billing needs.

You've got bills needing to be coded and sent in piling up. Have you made your decision?

This is where the biller will step in. They're going to perform their "initial scrub" at this step.

A reviewer at the third-party billing company is going to go through the file with a fine-tooth comb, essentially looking for a reason to say a "you're missing components" or "you can't bill for this."

While this sounds negative, it is actually a great thing! The scrubber is there to catch any snags in the process before they can put a wrench in the works. Essentially, the scrubber works as an accuracy checker for both any lapses in medical information and any incorrectly done billing. Their position is entirely checking off the box of "checks and balances."

From there, the biller will package everything up neatly in the patient's chart and ship it on to the appropriate insurance companies to be taken care of. They collect their fee for the service, sure, but they can also save your clinic and staff hours of time and anxiety spent in perfecting each bill.

NEGOTIATING YOUR FIRST CONTRACT

Initial negotiations can come in one of two ways.

1. Let's face it, individual specialty physicians are valuable because there's not enough of their specialty around. They'll give you a pretty good contract right off the bat to fill the gap they're facing.
2. On the other hand, insurance companies will look at you as if saying, "You know what? There are too many of your kind in this area. We're going to give you a half-assed contract." In this case, what they'll do is they pay you in different ways.

If you're in case number two, some of the insurance companies out there won't even bring you on their contract. "We don't need another right now!" This frequently happens in the world of primary care, internal medicine, family practice, and pediatrics. Alternatively, they may still take you on, but use this point in order to chip away at a much lower rate than usual.

There is a third way, though, but it requires a lot of work out of your own control:

3. If you're lucky and have enough patients with the same insurance company, ask to have you added into their coverage network, their insurance company may be pushed

to work with you or provide a better rate if they already do. Yes – in some ways, it is a popularity contest.

Know Medicare

At this stage, you've been asked to be on their insurance carrier. This is a great thing! However, you need to ask for at least 100% of what's called "Medicare Allowable Rate." Make a note here and underline, then highlight it.

While it is never talked about, insurance companies determine how much of their fee schedule, think of this as their "menu" of charges and what can be covered, based on Medicare payments.

Knowing this, essentially, the government is already dictating how much you're making because Medicare dictates your rates.

For example, a procedure that pays $500, let's say, in this case, an echocardiogram. The insurance company you're working with, a private insurance company, will come back and say to you, "We'll be paying you 90% of Medicare rates for a total of $450 for conducting this service."

While it seems like some number cruncher within the halls of their headquarters came up with that number, it isn't the case.

Medicare Allowable Rate – Ask for It!

Now you know the standard – this gives you power, as now you can negotiate with these insurance giants. Yes – it's possible!

Do your research. Let's say that you're one of the only physicians that do your specialty within 50 miles – this isn't uncommon! In this case, it isn't implausible to go back to the insurance company and ask for 130% compared to 100%.

On the other hand, if there are a number of doctors in your specialty in your area, the company may call back and offer, for example, an 80% rate. I've even seen it go as low as 60%!

You must understand your unique position and craft the angle to pursue in order to get a better rate - it can be a difficult battle to wage!

YOUR VALUES ARE YOUR BUSINESS

You're working hard to build your business and brand. You're seeing plenty of patients. Everything is going great.

There's still more work to be done!

You've got, at this point, what is called 'active income.' Active income means that you have to be actively involved in order to reap the rewards. AKA, you have to go into the office and see patients in order to make money and keep the office going.

Active income is the direct opposite of 'passive income' – as in interest on money in the bank, payouts from investments, royalties from book sales, rental income from properties you own, and other methods – you've probably picked up the difference – for passive income opportunities, they're 'set it and forget it.'

Start thinking about these options and gathering feasible ideas early. As you build your practice, you're building yourself a strong concrete foundation to build a skyscraper off of.

What's the big idea?

If you're looking to build your business, the secret is having multiple streams of income in place.

Risk Versus Reward – High Salaries

When a doctor such as a family doctor or internal medicine specialist looks at surgeons and plastic surgeons, there is often the unspoken question of: "Why do they make so much more money than me?" running through their minds.

The difference and defining factors are simple. A surgeon may wake up at two o'clock in the morning to immediately save a heart attack victim who is being wheeled in on the verge of death. Of course, that surgery could end in catastrophe, and then you could have multiple lawsuits and lose your reputation and potentially spiral into depression. This kind of work has high stakes around the clock.

Take that position versus you sitting in your office as a family physician, diagnosing colds and checking blood pressures until 5PM each day.

Just as in life, there is a lot of risk versus reward. The doctors with more challenging paths will bring home more at the end of the day – they're being paid for their training and expertise.

Doctor vs. 'The Hospital'

The hospital understands all this. They compensate, even overcompensate you, and do a good job of it. The only difference is you are not your own business. You're basically an employed or salaried physician. They give you a salary and tell you what to do.

You do what they say, and you earn your living, just like any other employee that's in that hospital – from the cleaning staff all the way up to the CEO. Given, there are benefits to this method! Surely, there is no shame in preferring this angle. If you like it, roll with it.

The Private Clinic Setting

In this setting, the client hires employees or new staff members directly, 'traditionally,' as you would say. This includes doctors, nurses, administrative staff, all the way down to the janitor.

Doctor salaries, of course, are much higher than the salaries of administrative staff, as an example. While you may pay administrators $15 an hour, you're looking at much, much more for a doctor.

A new physician, an interventional cardiologist, as an example, may cost you $750,000 a year.

With some simple math, you can determine how much you'll need to bring in to keep them. That's $62,500 a month. Quite a chunk of change out of your operating expenses, right?

The big question is: where is this money going to come from?

The harsh truth is that in the first few months, you'll lose money on their salary. This gap from hiring until the revenue comes in, where they "break even," is the amount of time that having them on the payroll will bring in patients, albeit from the outside, the doctor's own book of business, referrals, no matter what the mechanism may be.

Go down your list and check off each concern – almost like a "Yes/No" system. Once you've answered all the questions and you've reached the end – is the potential new hire worth it?

- Will they be able to bring in new business?
- Do they have a good track record of successfully treating patients?
- Do they bring their own book of business and patients with them?
- Do they have any outstanding issues, such as family problems?

Don't feel strange about it. In all honesty, this process is very similar to the process that all big sports firms go through when hiring an athlete, be it an NBA or an NFL player.

- "Does the player have a history of getting hurt?"
- "Is his personal life in order and out of the news?"

- "Did they have a great performance with their last team?"

Are you going to hire them?

What's the Pay Scale?

Your staff will do a lot and work plenty of hours. It's generally a better idea to overcompensate than undercompensate.

Let's face it, your staff are doing the nitty-gritty work. They're the ones that are the first line of defense. They're seeing your patients, cleaning your bathrooms, and doing your filing. When your patients walk in, you want them smiling, ready to help. If they're overstressed and underpaid – you aren't going to get that, no matter what.

Always overcompensate.

Always overvalue.

If you can't meet these two points with your current budget, then it is time to reevaluate and make changes to be able to do so.

Mitigating Risk

When we go on a date, we mitigate risk.

How do we do that?

We carry out our due diligence. We talk to our date frequently over the phone, by text, and by FaceTime. We look them up online and check everything out to make sure they are who they say they are. Then, when it's time for the first date, we meet up at a restaurant or bar – somewhere with other people around in case we have to hit the "escape" button.

It's the same thing when it comes down to medicine.

- When you're going to hire any staff member, especially a physician, you're going to do your entire due diligence. When you're hiring staff, you're going to do your due diligence on them. Do their references check out? Are their licenses good?
- When you're taking a risk and buying a building, you're going to mitigate your risks. You're going to offset your risk by doing your research on the location. As an example, sure, starting your clinic thirty minutes away from home, as compared to fifteen, may mean a cheaper rent on the space, but is the patient mix going to be different than it was closer to home? Are you going to be able to tolerate the additional drive back and forth? That's an extra thirty minutes! Coming home cranky every day will surely put a dampener on your family life. In this aspect, you're mitigating the risk of a divorce – the risks can be personal as well as professional. You're mitigating the risk of complications or problems at home. You're mitigating the risk of fatigue and burnout. It may end up that you decide the higher rent closer to home is worth the expense.

CHAPTER 4

WALKING THE BALANCE BEAM

"Are you not doing enough?"

That's a question that will stop most in their tracks and even offend some. That question is loaded with implied doubt.

What's your answer? Either way, how are you going to find balance?

CYCLES

The long, long hours required from the ground level up are an endless circle. At the minimum, you've put in 60 hours a week, all the way up to 140, all while trying to develop your own practice and doing your own business. You're working over a hundred hours a week, and try getting fewer hours in, and HR will be at your throat in a heartbeat.

What this means is that you're spending the night in the hospital. You're constantly waking up. There's not enough sleep to be had anywhere, guaranteed. You'll be woken up. More so, no matter what happens, you had better get used to it. You're in this hamster wheel to stay – you've paid out all this money for schooling and landed a job.

Welcome!

Where's the time for rest? Sleep? There's a little time in there, but there won't be much. In all of this, we commit a capital crime against ourselves – we forget that we exist as human beings.

In this state of forgetting, there is no balance in the beginning. You are basically sacrificing your body, your mind, your mental state for the benefit of helping others and making it in the medical profession.

Recovering While in the Hamster Wheel

It was my first year, I was working nearly nonstop. A call for a STEMI came in – a heart attack – these are frequent, and you can get called in at any time of the night if a doctor who can handle them isn't on the schedule.

It was two-thirty in the morning when my beeper rang – we were still using those back then, not too long ago! I had been asleep, for, at maximum, thirty minutes, and I was so tired that it took me an extra minute to find my beeper, even though it was only on the nightstand right next to my bed.

This may sound like an exaggeration, but it isn't – a truck driver fell over with a heart attack at a 24-hour McDonald's after eating two big macs. The ambulance crew lifted him off the floor and took him straight to the hospital.

By the time I get to him, he's nearly gone. We do the procedure, and he makes it. From there, he's put on a ventilator for a couple of weeks. However, when you're put on a ventilator, you're also put into a medical coma.

After a few weeks, he's taken off the ventilator and brought back to an awake state – I go back to see him. Outside of the nurse, maybe, if he was awake, I was probably the first person to truly talk to him in weeks.

The situation started out normally as I came in; he wearily looked over and went, "Who are you?"

Exuding my usual bedside manner, I approach, assuring him. "I'm your doctor – I did your heart surgery; I saved your life."

The man thought for a few seconds, let out a deep breath, and almost rolled his eyes, "Can you get me a cigarette?"

While that moment is shocking, sure, it was also an intense learning moment, almost like a turning point. You're saving someone's life, sure, but in a way, you're working for the patient – a patient that may turn around and undo everything that you worked to save them from. Knowing that patient, I'm sure the first night back on the road, he stopped in for a burger and had a few cigarettes. It's a tough thing to think about.

Your clients are going to make their own choices. You can't hold their hands and make their decisions for them. Knowing this, you've got to prioritize yourself; you've got to think about yourself and take a break.

Maybe it's better not to work that many hours and to take some time off – maybe you don't do those 24-hour call times. Sure, the building up of your career will take a little longer, but will the benefits be worth it? The effects of this decision will build up over time – it may be later, maybe even years, but you'll see the difference between yourself and those in your professional circle that never took time for themselves – they may be a little richer, sure, but are they put together?

Return of the 30 Minute Break

A clear mind, body, and spirit lead to well-planned decisions. Without these essential elements in place, you might as well be going into work drunk.

Most doctors spend ten to fifteen years growing into their

eventual position. If you spend an extra thirty minutes a day, at least fifteen, focusing on one other item, whatever that may be, as long as it is practical, you can be successful at that other item at the same time. You can be successful at being a physician and as a professional in another field as well.

For example, let's talk about real estate. If you spend 30 minutes a day learning about EBITDA, administration of real estate, mortgages, cap rates, zoning, and taxes, your priorities on finding locations for purchase suddenly become easier to handle in the few hours you have each week for it.

These small lessons will pay off for you later in the future; in this case, there's no head-scratching when it comes down to business decisions around offices. There's no need to pay a realtor commission, bringing on an expensive lawyer, or regretting decisions later.

Get Exercise

Maybe you're not exercising. Maybe you're not doing your daily meditation. If you're not, there's no peace of mind to be had.

- You're not likely to make good decisions in anything you do.
- Maybe you're going to have bad outcomes in your personal life.
- Maybe you're going to have bad surgical outcomes.
- Maybe you're going to have bad patient outcomes.
- No outcome will be the best version of itself.

FINDING SANITY

Let's use an example of two made-up doctors.

The first doctor is going through financial troubles, his house is in danger of being foreclosed, and he's having marital issues. He's called in for an emergency case, an intervention case – he's got a patient that needs a stent placed for a heart catheterization. These emergencies are relatively common but can get complicated quickly with unknown elements.

The doctor starts but hits a complication fairly quickly – this patient's blood vessels are dense, and it is taking a little longer to gain access. The patient starts to crash – it is time to move quickly, or they'll likely die.

The code blue is called out, but no other doctors are able to help – he freezes, stands there with his arms folded, and cannot make a decision. No idea what to do. Everyone in the room stands over the opened patient, looking at the doctor with a look of "Well, what do we do now?"

The problem is that the doctor has no idea what to do. He can't do anything. The mental anguish has gotten to him and stopped his mind from working – it is now dead cold. He is unable to now fulfill his obligations as a surgeon, and I've seen it firsthand. The best case in this scenario is that another doctor can take over – at worst, the patient dies and now both doctors have grief.

The ability to make important decisions starts with being able to take care of yourself.

The Biological Basis

Most studies say that we only use 20% of our brain's "computing power." You're probably using a little bit more if you're taking care of yourself, but you need to maximize that potential. You need to expand your knowledge. You know, being a doctor is no excuse to just know medicine only.

Interestingly, this idea translates into managing your assets.

Understanding the Job's Emotional Toll

How do you refuel? How do you access empathy?

It's an interesting question and one that doctors must know the answer to ahead of time – to make things even more complicated, the answer is unique for everyone, just as unique as our own fingerprints.

With a stockbroker, you have the highs and lows when a stock goes up and down – it's a factor of excitement when stocks are up and depression when stocks are down, but until you sell, you aren't really losing anything. Medicine is a little different.

For example, I had a case where I was seeing a patient fairly early in my career, about a year in. She was this little old lady, having chest pain, the first patient of the morning. I start a heart catheterization, as is normal procedure. She goes through, comes off the medicine, and she's just fine – alert and talking to us, no problems.

In the waiting room, she crashes and passes away – seemingly out of the blue.

At the end of the day, it was an allergic reaction. Something that none of us could have predicted, she never showed any signs of an allergy.

I wept like a little baby. I cried. I almost hung up my white coat for good.

Every doctor has this first-time experience. From that first case on, your mental state now changes for every single patient that comes in through the doors to see you – emergency or not. You're thinking about every single scenario now where that can happen again to you. The problem is that if that thinking gets out of control, it can freeze you – an allergy can hit anyone. Young or old.

For the next four weeks, I was not the same person – I couldn't help but feel death lingering around all of my patients – even though I wasn't personally responsible, I felt that I was.

What a way to see more patients – feeling like you've been beaten up and ready to bleed out – really, your soul feels broken. You have families that get involved with you, and they're very close to you. What do you do when things fall through? How do you tell them?

I once had a case with a husband and wife – I was handling the wife. When they were younger, they would go fishing together. They were good friends. Of course, as they grew up, they fell in love and got married.

They had a great relationship – the husband was known for randomly giving her presents. They truly were great role models. Even though I was handling only his wife, the husband would always come in with her. He was a good friend with political figures and always had great stories.

The first time she ever came to meet with me without him, of course, I asked where he was – that's when she had to tell me that he had died. I knew he'd had pancreatic cancer, but we all thought he would beat it. He left a trinket for me; it was a fishing lure from JFK. His wife gave it to me and told me, he would want you to have this. Cherish it like he did.

It can happen to any of us.

Overcoming the Lows

What's your purpose? Why is it so important that you are in the field of medicine and that you're caring for humanity?

Most physicians get into the field because they enjoy taking care of someone; that's the truth. However, let's think of this a little deeper.

When a doctor takes care of a patient, everybody thinks that he's doing it to help that patient, but there is an aspect of mental greed; the doctor's also doing it for himself because he feels good about

69

it – and of course, the paychecks are good. The doctor comes out of it feeling good too.

What does that tell you about the doctor's ego and his brain? What is the real purpose?

Of course, we're all meeting the means to an end, but, again, doctors are human beings as well – there's nobody out there who doesn't scratch their own back when helping someone else. It is a hard truth to swallow and understand, but an essential one.

Going a little deeper, there are very few fields in medicine that actually save lives. Most of the fields are "preventative medicine," which can really be translated into "prolonging or improving life." You're not really saving it unless you're handling cancer, heart attacks, lung problems, and brain tumors as examples.

Take a step back as a physician, as a medical student, as a nurse, any position you may be filling. Ask yourself two questions:

1. Are you prolonging someone's life with your actions?
2. Are you doing your job to make yourself happy or truly help your patient, saving their life or improving their life's quality?

If that's the case, then you should be doing the same thing for yourself. You need to have a good quality of life for yourself as well. Remind yourself why you're in medicine with those two questions.

OUTSIDE THE OFFICE

You've barely got a moment at home! That's what the proverbial hamster wheel feels like. You know, the days turn into weeks, weeks to months, months to years. And before, you know, it, life is flying by.

AT HOME

You can't let your home life go.

Growing Expenditures

It comes true for everyone in a position with a higher income than the national average. Particularly in the top 25%, where doctors with specialties are often lumped in, even the ones who work in typical hospital systems.

That money piles up and goes to your head. The houses get a little larger. Car purchases get fancier and more frequent. Suddenly there's a boat and a dock in the backyard. Every luxury you can think of makes it in through the front door.

Nobody stops to think about what's really happening – that the credit card needs to be put down – by then, it is too late. A precedent has already been set within your family and relationships. Bigger is better.

All of a sudden, the bank account that was once more than enough starts to suffer hits. The expenditures get a little 'braver,' taking out large chunks at a time. Your wife, who may have had an element of spendthrift when you were a resident, is now buying a Chanel purse once a month. Your kids are always getting new cell phones because they carelessly break their old ones, forgetting the days when they had to take proper care of them. Your car goes from a sensible BMW to a Ferrari or Lamborghini.

All of a sudden, you need to spend more than 90 hours at the office to even keep your bank account at a safe baseline. Try asking your family to cut back? Good luck.

Do You lack in the Communication Department?

You've got luxuries, and if the costs are in check, even better. You've got opportunities in life to experience the world and the heights of your career. Great! You've probably got a contact list full of all types of great relationships and a family that loves you.

I've been there, done it, and got the t-shirt.

All of this isolated work in your bubble, though, will probably start to do a number on your communication skills – talking to your wife is much different than shouting out orders and moves during a code blue.

It is easy to transfer the stress of a heart attack case from earlier in the day to see to it that the kitchen is clean after making dinner. Suddenly, that heart attack case escalates some spilled sauce onto the counter into an argument about an entire marriage.

On the flip side, you've spent your entire day at the hospital negotiating a salary increase with HR and are totally exhausted by the time you get home – "I don't care what we have for dinner, just order a pizza or something." While it isn't your fault that you're exhausted, that is human. Suddenly, you've pulled yourself from even the most basic choices and decisions in family life – you begin to become a shadow. The problem is that, in this case, the only time you do react will be when you're angry or stressed. You become not just a shadow, but an angry presence – you'll begin to be avoided.

You've set your path to learning about your niche interests, sure, but there's another set of factoids that you need to know even better – your own family. What are your partner's dislikes and likes? What is the name of your kid's school? When's their birthday? Their favorite meal?

If you don't talk to your partner for a month about work, and then all of a sudden, you come home and say, "Listen, I had a patient that really did poorly, and I'm sad." Your partner is going to have no frame of reference. I'll tell you what they'll be thinking.

"Where did this come from? I don't understand. Now you're taking it out on our family and everybody else and moping around like a dope."

It's critically important that there's communication now, decide how much you're going to share – I'll always be an advocate for as much as possible. From there, you and your partner have to understand that each of your contributions are going to be different from the discussion but come together as a whole. Sometimes, despite what you've ever been told, it is a good idea to take your work home.

Misunderstandings are bound to happen along the way with even the most well-connected of spouses. There will come a time when you're overbooked and have to stay at work late. How do you deal with those sacrifices when coming back home?

It's not just the clear communication, as we mentioned earlier, but it's also the aspect of making an effort, because what happens when you're tired, you've done a 17-hour day, and you're coming home, and all you want to do is eat and go to sleep?

Your kids are still going to be running around when you get home; they're young, they don't understand how tired you are – once you get them settled down, you've got your partner asking for private time. None of that is work-related, but they are obligations to fulfill. They're the second hemisphere of your world.

What's more is that it doesn't end at your front door. It's your friends outside of home. How do you keep your relationship with the boys or girls group up? Whether you're a doctor, a surgeon, or a nurse, it is critical to have non-work friends.

Putting a Cap on Jealousy

Picture this – me, a solo doctor, just coming out of medical school – bright-eyed and bushy-tailed, as the saying goes. I was very skillfully trained in my training, went to quite a few fellowships, and did some special training even further outside – that meant I had targets on my back.

There are two aspects to this:

1. You're jealous of someone.
2. That someone is jealous of you.

Seems deceptive, almost childishly simple, right?

In the aspect of the jealousy ingredient, you have to take a step back. You have to think about what your purpose really is – are you going to spend the energy you have, which you can't get back or more of, to go after someone, or deal with their blows and continue trekking on?

It is smarter to simply continue doing your own thing. You're getting hammered, and you have the target on your back. It is very important that you do not make mistakes at that time – all eyes are on you, and someone is looking for any tiny failure to begin the process of trying to get rid of you. I've seen it happen to many doctors in many settings – usually unjustly so.

There's envy anywhere that money is involved; we know this. When you start eating up the market share of an area, putting up office after office, and poaching great talent, it will be noticed. It doesn't end outside of the office, though.

No matter what type of doctor you are, no matter what type of specialist, no matter what type of surgeon, you'll wind up going to functions where there are other doctors, their families, and their associates – these are important, as that's where you build your contact base. However, there's always an element of jealousy there, even if it is only jealousy that we create based on outside assumptions, which we know generally aren't true.

— *"Are they a better surgeon?"*
— *"Was that the person driving a Maserati?"*

— *"How in the hell is their practice bigger than mine?"*
— *"I bet he's loaded."*

Immediate envy.

We Aren't Living in An Action Movie

Not everyone is out directly competing against you. If you're a heart surgeon, there isn't a lot of reason to be anxious over the intentions of a regular family doctor, for example. They can refer cases to you, sure, but they surely can't unseat your position – they don't have the skills or tools to do so. To fear them would be to create generalized anxiety, which isn't good for anyone.

Manage Your Own Social Book

It's up to you to manage your own relationships.

Personally, I always chose to keep my relationships outside of work fairly close and small – generally family and the parents of the kids that my own children went to school with.

There's a term for this – 'finding your tribe.'

That sentiment may sound silly, but it represents a great idea – find a group of individuals that support you and welcome you into their fold. You want to feel included. We're social creatures as human beings, after all. Now, you can be part of a few different tribes, such as personal and business – but those tribes must be close-knit.

Aside from belonging socially, there's another social aspect that they play a hand in – they keep you responsible to your tribe. You have to put the time in. A tribe doesn't allow you to be sucked into only work and become a shadow. They'll help you to regulate your time – although it is still your duty to heed their concerns.

You can be yourself; you don't have to play-act to belong in a group. Work until you find the few permanent members of your tribe, then let the others come and go.

SELF-CARE

The most prominent example of lack of self-care in medicine is never having time to eat. That beeper or cell phone goes off, and you are dropping your sandwich, and that's even if you get a moment to sit down. At best, in most levels of medicine, we get a pause for fifteen minutes every few hours, and that pause could be standing up or doing something else, just a little bit slower.

Not exactly components that create a healthy lifestyle.

Create a Schedule

What makes this topic easy is that there are hundreds of ready-to-use formats online to simply fill in – there's no excuse to not do this today. Have a schedule that doesn't only accommodate work but also involves mind, body, and spirit. A schedule that puts you into the groove of a healthy lifestyle. What that means is you can't just eat these garbage breakfast and lunches just because you have no time – your schedule tells you when and how much time you have.

You're In the Health Business… Stay Healthy!

Neglect the healthy aspects of your lifestyle, and your brainpower is going to suffer, not to mention your entire body.

A great example of this is the classic "drug rep dinner." These are extremely common and go on beneath patients' noses. These events are invitation-only dinners, usually at a fancy restaurant or hotel ballroom, depending on how many invites are sent out, held by pharmaceutical manufacturers. During the dinner, speakers from the company, including doctors, but really, salesmen, present the latest drugs on offer and their benefits. It really can be a snake oil show. The ultimate aim of these dinners is to onboard you to use their medicines or devices. The way that they draw doctors in is offering a free dinner – usually whatever you want from a broad, fully-expanded menu.

The famous food critic Anthony Bourdain said in a famous video that in most restaurants of higher quality, you leave having eaten at least two sticks of butter. It's true.

Doctors start to put on weight because, if you really wanted to, you could find one of these drug rep dinners nearly every night. That's going on at least six to eight sticks of butter a week if you eat an average meal.

Add on free alcohol, and you're looking at liver disease territory.

Fat, fat, fat - because when it's free, you order whatever you want. There's no shame in this. It's natural; it's what people do in life. However, if you slow down and stop for a second and say, "You know what, I can't go to that drug dinner because I would rather enjoy spending that time with my family," things start to change.

Read Up, Learn, Watch, Experience

Personally, and I'm sure it is the same for many others, I'd rather enjoy that time, that hour or two to myself, by going to the gym or reading a book, catching up on the news, or learning about my own niche: interest, stocks, and investments. My broker would call me every few months and say, "You're missing out on all the moments to pounce; you're so busy. Do you want to sell and just get out?"

The man had a point, I have to admit. I would just think of him and talk to him at the end of the year and see what my numbers were. My investments simply weren't something I was going to put active time towards.

Suddenly, though, putting time into my schedule for investments after that call, I do my reading. I can already see the entire growth because now I read up on market changes – most of the time, I call my broker before he calls me in order to make changes and take advantage of the market.

You Need Sleep, But Do So With Reason

I've always had a philosophy in life – that sleep is a waste of time.

I can be doing things in the middle of the night – even better, with less distraction – everyone else is asleep! Even today, I use the night to create and write down new ideas before I get my few hours in – the amount that my body needs, but no more.

Everyone lives by the six-to-eight-hour rule. That's what we're all taught. There have been studies that cast some doubt on the idea, but most science supports it. It is true that some of us require more sleep, so there's no cut-and-dried rule here. However, the idea is to pack our days and schedule them out so that those six to eight hours of sleeping aren't truly lost; they're simply a means to an end.

Make time to prioritize your time because the world won't do it for you.

A WORD ON BURNOUT

Burnout can hit at random times and in ways that we can never predict before it springs up. We can start to lose interest in our family, our work, our friends, find our health declining, and many other factors. In a way, burnout causes our anxieties to come true – a term you may have heard before, a 'self-fulfilling prophecy.' We put so much energy and mental anguish into mindsets that it finds a way to make them happen – when in fact, our minds have been psychologically pushing us toward them. There's no magic to it.

Connect with those people outside of your respective industry—your family, friends, and loved ones. Again, build yourself a schedule that tells you when you should pursue these activities – it will cut out any potential heartaches of not finding the time.

"You are your own person, your own business, and you'll find a way to be successful, but you also have to find ways to help yourself." If you take care of yourself more, those wise decisions and your inner voice will be that much clearer and that much stronger. We can put back out what we put in.

For doctors, burnout is that voice in the back of your head that's saying, "You're falling behind. You need to make sure you get caught up; you're ahead of the game."

What do you say to that voice in this same conversation of making sure that you're carving out time that could be spent working on X, Y, and Z at the office, but you know that you need to take some time out for yourself?

"It needs to be done."

When you do that, you're anticipating things, and that's the way it should be. If you're not going to anticipate what's going to happen for the next 10 hours, and you're not able to plan, you will feel like you're falling behind constantly because you don't know what to expect.

Let's face it, when you're falling behind, it changes your entire mental state, but I'm going to tell you, when you feel like you're falling behind, you need to say one important thing.

"#*ck it!" That's it.

CHAPTER 5

THE BIG THREE

We're switching over to business mode here; we're talking stocks and cryptocurrency, ETFs, mutual stocks, bonds, and establishing a business or two or three. No worries here – we're doctors, not business brokers or bankers, but we know enough to operate in each realm we invest our time because we spend our allotted 'me time' wisely.

I. BUSINESS

Most physicians are only in one of these categories, business usually being the one they're primarily invested in. You've got your clinic, or maybe you're looking to grow out of a health system and roll into your own clinic. From there, what other support businesses can you develop?

II. PERSONAL DEVELOPMENT

You are the source of your business' income! After all, patients aren't paying to come in and check out the waiting room. You develop alongside your businesses individually.

My daughter, when she was little, asked me point blank, "What grade are you when you finish becoming a cardiologist?"

That question took me back for a second, but I had to be honest. "I'm 32nd grade." (My age at the time!)

III. ARMS-LENGTH ACHIEVEMENTS

What are arms-length achievements? In short, they're short, effective achievements that you can take on and accomplish rather quickly – think of them as daily victories.

You've got a limited number of hours in a day. You've got to see patients, you've got to see your family when you get home, and then you've got your sleeping, eating, driving, etc. – the basics of human life.

What you're doing is limiting yourself – what's the limit?

Your income is limited by the percentage you can be physically present, such as seeing patients. Sure, this can be done through telehealth to some extent, but it still requires your physical presence on the other end of the line. It isn't time's fault; it is a fault that we all have – that we can't be everywhere at once. Every time you take care of yourself, you've checked off an arms-length achievement.

THE ELEMENTS OF THE BIG THREE

Five unique elements go under the umbrella of 'the big three,' which build them into how important they truly are:

1) **Expand your vision**

2) **Be passionate**

3) **Find your own ventures**

4) **Find expert opinions**

5) **Execute your plan**

1) <u>Expand Your Vision</u>

You know what your goal is: to expand so that incomes are flowing in from other sources while you're attending to your office, your family, or yourself.

There's a word for this, and you've likely heard it. "Passive income."

Now, this passive income could be just about anything as long as it is generating positive cash flow. It could be rent from real estate investments, gains on stocks, or appreciating values of cryptocurrencies you're holding onto.

For example, let's say you've got a medical supply industry where you've got a buildup – clients and connections leading to a profit. That's passive income in one little sentence.

A Personal Story: Playing the Cards Right

When I was 13 years old, there was a desirable baseball card. In particular, it was for Ken Griffey Jr. He had a baseball card in 1989, an Upper Deck™ one, to be precise. The card was quite collectible and not impossible to come by. It was one of those strange outliers in the card market that always had value and would spike occasionally. (That's right – I was hustling even then.)

I would buy his card, and then I would sell the card for a higher profit, even if it was five bucks, or ten bucks – maybe not a huge price hike but remember the cost of packs of cards at the time – if I invested every cent in that sale, I could walk away with up to twenty new packs!

Obviously, any time I could get my hands on that Ken Griffey Jr. card, I would snatch it up as quickly as I could – I knew that card would always make me money. After all, baseball cards are interesting in that even today, when the player on the card does well, the value of his card goes up. He was obviously a good player!

A Personal Story: Working the Circuit

I always thought about having multiple jobs, even when I was young. I would work at Long John Silver's®, even during the school year, walking my way there every weekend after cramming my homework in.

During the summer, I would pick up a second job at the supermarket chain Winn-Dixie, where I worked in the seafood department. (They were keen on giving me that position due to my time at Long John Silver's®!)

Sometimes in college, I would try to schedule my shifts while I was in between classes, but my whole goal was multiple sources of income. With that extra cash in my pocket, I would invest it in other ventures.

2) Be passionate

With your own practice, acting on your own accord, you're in charge. You're making the last decision when you're seeing the patient and the last decision when signing off on purchase orders for boxes of gauze. Are you going to spend an extra hour with that patient for an additional test or upgrade the gauze to a brand that is a little more absorbent? It's all yours to decide. That falls onto the bigger decisions as well, whether you're hiring staff, firing staff, or expanding your offices.

When purchasing a property, there's always a commission involved for someone, whether it be your independent realtor or their brokerage firm.

"They aren't doing anything special; I could be keeping that commission for myself."

I can't help but remember the moment that line flashed through my mind, having just signed on the line for a new office space – the realtor was ecstatic, of course. Florida real estate is never cheap!

As a result, I thought to myself. "Why couldn't I do this?" I started getting defensive! I mean, at that moment, I was feeling like a real dope for handing over a wad of cash that I didn't necessarily have to give away.

Arms-length, a passive income opportunity. That's it.

"Why can I not do this? I've gone to school; I'm 32 years old. There's no indication that I'm not smart enough to do it. Why shouldn't I be able to study what a brokerage is and then open up my own brokerage firm so that I can keep my own money?" I was going to save myself a very large chunk of change, that is true, but I also wanted to prove to myself that I could do it.

Under real estate, there are multiple opportunities right under your nose, whether it's residential, which we're all beyond familiar with, and then there's commercial, like retail or office space. There's one more category, though, brokerage – one that most of us never utilize.

In our example, healthcare brokerage, you're still purchasing and selling properties for the sake of creating offices to utilize and rent out to other doctors. Essentially, you're acting as your own personal real estate agent and developer, all wrapped up into one.

Let me be honest. At first, it's overwhelming –

"I don't understand what these are."
"I don't know if I can understand what capital gains are."
"I have no clue what unrealized gain or loss is."
"What's shorting a stock?"

"I might not know now, so it is time to dive in and start studying."

3) Find Your Own Ventures

I used the same concept that I always followed – to dive in and start studying. The medical supplies were the same concept. I'm buying from a third party, who's marking it up 10 to 15%. Why not go straight to the wholesaler and purchase these medical supplies for myself? Most suppliers, even today, only require you to show some basic licensure you already have on hand to create an account.

From there, it began to feel like a Costco or Sam's Club operation – I connected with other healthcare offices to grow my orders into larger bulk purchases, getting a deeper and deeper discount. It's sort of like running an old-fashioned general store.

What's the worst-case scenario? You lose a little money if it doesn't work out, and you go back to the old way of doing things. Sure, that part, quite frankly, sucks, but it's really interesting. Your passion translated to a variety of different interests as well as business opportunities for that passive income.

In this hypothesized example, you work in a hospital system: you put in a heart stent for a patient, and you've earned your paycheck, great! However, as we know, the hospital has made three times the amount from charging the patient's insurance.

Of course, the patient needs to stay in for a few days for recovery and monitoring – making the hospital a grand amount of up to $120,000 for that patient to be there for a couple of days before they go on home. Through this time, you, as the doctor, are making some money as well, seeing over the patient's case. By the end, you've likely pocketed anywhere from $500-$3,000.

Let's do a little math.

$120,000 - $3,000 = $117,000.

That's right, the hospital made $117,000 on the work that you, as the doctor, provided. The CEO and investors surely weren't in the room! Sweet deal for them, huh?

I went to an insurance company, Blue Cross Blue Shield, one of the largest and highest-utilized in the United States. "I'm going to build my own surgical center, and I'm going to do this procedure in our office. Will you guys be willing to help us to do this together?"

What was their response? To paraphrase, it was "of course!"

Why would they agree? Easy. To them, they're saving a large amount of money not paying into the hospital system, bar none. While I'm able to charge a handsome fee at my own clinic, the fee is going to be low enough to be extremely attractive to insurance companies – plus, your clinic won't be charging various hospital administration fees; not to mention the fact that the insurance company will be able to funnel more patients your way, as your services are just as good quality while being more affordable. Access to care widens for patients, and your pool of potential clients grows exponentially in markets where doctors of your type are hard to come by.

The best part of it all? This entire process is "street legal" – it follows all state and federal health guidelines – as long as your clinic is clean, safe, and efficient, you're on board to succeed. Knowing this, that regulations are in place, the marketplace is wide open – private insurance carriers and even Medicare are potential sources of partnerships. In the United States, politicians love good old-fashioned capitalism, and, at bare bones, that's what this concept is.

A Personal Story: The Timeshare Anecdote

The concept of the timeshare came when I built my first surgery center. I didn't have much income at that point, but I took a risk in building it. Some would say that the idea was one born of necessity – sometimes the best ones!

When the surgery center was completed, I now had a number of unused slots on my hands that could take on doctors and patients – it was only me at the time, but I had predicted a growing clinic of more doctors. It was just a matter of time. Don't get me wrong though, I wanted that 'time' to be as short as possible – those empty spots were costing me!

The big kicker is that I was in that office one day a week. I sat and thought to myself, "You know what? Other doctors are going to want to use this. I live in the timeshare capital of the world, which is Orlando, Florida. There's got to be some way to work with that idea."

To be honest, I didn't know what a "timeshare" was before I moved to Florida, just as you may not, but I'll break it down simply – for a yearly fee, paid out no matter what way, the person paying into a timeshare, in exchange, is given "X" amount of time each year to spend at the property. For example, you may pay $2,000 a year for a full week's worth of time at a beachside condo. For all the other weeks out of the year, others who are paying in are able to utilize the condo.

I hit the books. I talked with real estate professionals.

I applied the same concept, renting out the spaces, and sometimes the full facility, to doctors. They would bring in their own staff, do their own billing, and run the facility as their own except I would be the landlord, taking on the typical responsibility of repairs and cleanliness – even better, as these doctors were essentially 'traveling,' I also sold them medical supplies from my own supply company within the building.

4) <u>Find Expert Opinions</u>

My philosophy has always been simple. You don't have to be the smartest person in the room – that's complicated. *You want to be as smart as you can be, but you want to surround yourself with other smart individuals who know about the field you're exploring.* Now, that's much simpler – you're acting as a human rather than a memory bank.

Now, if I spent twenty minutes a day reading about how to set up a medical supply company, for example, as I did, I'm going to be much more equipped to make solid financial and business decisions. That knowledge, a solid investment, has kept me from going into additional debt or taking on additional costs through having to pay a distributor, who marks up their prices, to get my medical supplies into the office.

Let's look at another angle, knowing how to set up the administration for a Cardiac PET scanner, rather than taking on the cost of a specially-trained staff member or consultant to set up and maintain the system. Sure, if I can't find enough information on my own, I may talk to an expert, then do my own research from what they suggest – either way, I'm learning on my own.

Time equals money, even when it is coming in. This isn't a concept that only applies to money going out!

When your financial advisor comes to you and gives you

advice on a stock, yes, you take the advice, you review the advice. But this is where it makes a difference. You go and do research on your own, and you may agree or disagree with them, whether it's Apple stock or a penny stock in some brand-new startup. They're all important.

A Personal Story: You're – Not So Full of It...

Sometimes, those strange ideas pitched to you out of the middle of nowhere aren't so strange at all.

Pre-med school: That feels like a lifetime ago now. I had a friend who was on the business track. He had a project and was trying to avoid working on it. I was working at the computer lab at the time as a monitor while he came in every day to try and get the project done when not goofing off.

One afternoon, I finally walked over and asked what he was doing, seeing the lists of stocks go by on that blue and black screen. "I'm working on a project where we've got to build fake stocks, and we see how they do. We watch them over six months, and some of us actually invest in those that are close to how our projects perform, using them kind of like an indicator."

I look at him kind of strangely because it was a rather strange project, but it seems feasible – the reasoning is there, after all. He looks at me with the same amused enthusiasm. "You need to invest in this stock. It's really big. It's going to become huge."

Following his advice and consulting with him, I started investing in stocks and mutual funds and just letting the money grow. Looking back, I wish I could have done even more. The hustle that I had back then when I was in my early medical career, because I had a lot more money at that time, well, money I could freely spend.

This didn't mean that I was infallible, though.

The time was somewhere in the late '90s. The 'dot.com bubble' was growing with the internet beginning to come in at full force. I continued seeing my friend come in each afternoon, and I start gaining true interest in his project.

A few weeks in, he shows me a name on the computer of a real company that is having a bumpy time of it but seems to be showing real progress.

"It doesn't sound serious to me," I remember saying to my friend, looking at the name of the business, "It sounds childish. They aren't going to go very far."

My friend practically begged me to invest. "Just one or two stocks!"

While I did nothing, my friend tossed in the spare cash he had to buy some stock in the growing company. You're probably guessing what the company could have been.

It was the classic decoration on schoolteachers' desks around the country. Apple!

Listen to everyone. If they give you advice, go research it on your own and look it up and figure it out.

5) Execute your plan

If you're thinking about doing something, whether it's outside the realm or scope of your practice or business, you've already taken the first step by following through on that idea floating in your head. The second step is to understand it and do your research. *The third step, and the most important, is to execute your plan.*

Whatever it may be in life, whether it's thinking about getting married, having children, working on a home improvement project, buying a new property, expanding your business, going back to school, or going on a date, if it's an idea, it's time to execute.

You don't want to have regrets on your deathbed.

If you don't try anything, it's worse than trying and failing.

CHAPTER 6

HOW THE COGS COME TOGETHER

Looking at the hospital system from a wide-angle lens, we can think of it as a factory that pumps out patients. No matter their outcomes – their case may be resolved, or it may not. Inside of that factory, there is specialty equipment and trained staff to see everything through to the end, just like in a factory.

As students, we tend to think that we'll do medical school, take on a residency, then be a doctor – bam! It isn't that easy though, there's a system to go through, molds to fit on the production line until we reach the end.

Let's face it, while you're going through this, you really don't see the administrative side. You don't see the financial side of it. You're basically a pawn, for lack of a better word, in the health system. Remember, you're making money for the hospital system's pocket and keeping your little percentage at the end.

Everyone plays their role to make the 'clock' tick, even the parts under the hood that you don't see, from the pharmacy to finance and HR. Let's start by looking at the rungs of the ladder you'll have to climb on the way to becoming a doctor at large.

Internships 101

You've graduated from medical school; that's a great step! There's still more to go, though; you've got to go out in the world, get hands-on experience, and prove yourself as an up-and-coming doctor. You're now a doctor, sure, you've got the degree, but there isn't a patient in the world who is going to let a book-smart world-untested doctor perform their surgery alone.

They wear white coats. You've seen them. As an intern, you'll be called to do a little bit of everything. At this stage, your specialty doesn't matter as much. You could be stitching up a wound in the ER all the way up to assisting in surgery. It's all in the name of preparing to face the unknown on your own.

A Personal Story: Impromptu OB/GYN

Going back to my intern years, I'm on call and am quickly called up to the medical floor for a strange case. The nurse, trying to be delicate about it, catches me on the way up and explains that it's a 22-year-old female with bleeding issues. This complaint is relatively routine, sure; however, I'm training to become a cardiologist, not an OB/GYN.

It's 11 in the evening, and I'm seeing over an intimate bleeding case. Always the unexpected. I enter the "cubicle" to find the patient and her boyfriend lying down in her patient bed. After introductions, I ask her if she'll be able to manage until in the morning when the OB/GYN staff arrives – she agrees; I wish her the best, prescribe some Tylenol, and tell them to hold off.

At 2:00 am, I'm called back into the room – she's having more severe pain at this point.

I go through the entire diagnostic checklist, checking off each box as I go along; everything seems to be fairly standard; in the end, I concluded that this could likely be a routine complaint that simply was built up to get out of hand, but it is time to continue with the more professional exam. The nurse to accompany me arrives, and we begin, asking the boyfriend to leave the room.

Within seconds of examining her, I discovered the issue. A lodged tampon.

That's when the truth was revealed. She had sex with her boyfriend while the tampon was stuck in her vaginal canal, pushing it deeper in and lacerating her uterus. As a result, we had to call her in for surgery. Of course, she was stitched up and came out just fine, but that's the life of an intern; it's not about your specialty; it's what's thrown at you. You expect someone to know that it's common sense not to have sex with a tampon inserted, but sure, it happens.

A Personal Story: Surgical Concerns

An early-morning car crash survivor came in, and on intake was put on the list for surgery that day. To tide the patient over until time, they were put onto a direct IV drip of morphine to regulate their pain – standard operating procedure. It was 5:00 AM, and I was on pre-surgery patient rounds, just the collection of generic information and to get to know the patient. In this case, I was lucky to have the surgeon with me as well. As we completed our discussions, we noticed that the IV equipment beeped warnings continuously and it could be heard outside the patient's room. Once we completed the interview, I went back in to figure out why the equipment was continuing to beep.

Within a minute, I figured out the source and the reason why. One of her family members was sitting so close to the equipment – they'd unplugged the IV drip and were sucking on the morphine, leaving their hurt family member high and dry.

The strangest things will happen. It isn't a chance, it will. The likelihood of shenanigans also extends to your patient, their families, friends, and visitors.

A Personal Story: Orthopedics

Imagine this: I'm an intern on a rotation for orthopedics. Quite different from cardiology, huh, dealing with bones?

At the time, we're sitting in for the morning report, all of the orthopedic residents and chief orthopedic resident gathered around, taking in the news about each case on the ward. However, this morning, we're interrupted by a code blue on the overhead speaker, causing the entire room to jump to attention. Someone in the hospital was dying, and immediate help is needed. One of us needs to charge out and assist, but the head resident stops me with just one question.

"Does anyone in this room have a stethoscope on them?"

No. We are orthopedic surgery residents, far from the heart and vascular system. No one had one. Lesson learned; Understand your role and limits.

A Personal Story: Accountability

I know there are many "above all else" statements to be said about the early years, but here's another. Above all else, be on time.

I can't help but remember one of my fellow interns, in the early days, showing up around one minute late – no more. They were told to go home for the rest of the day. "Go home, think it over. You don't want to be here."

You could've cut the tension with the edge of a piece of paper at that moment. I've never forgotten it – I can play it through my mind like a movie on demand. I suppose it is a story of being on time, but also one of a reminder – know that you want to be there.

Residency 101

After the intern stage, your residency coat gets a little longer, both literally and figuratively. Even so, from there, there are a few levels of residents. There's the second-year resident, third-year resident, then the chief resident, essentially the fourth-year. As a fourth-year chief resident, you're expected to act with autonomy and make no mistakes; in a lot of ways, you're a full-fledged doctor without the title. It's insulting in a way, yes, but the hospital system is doing this to cover themselves should you make a mistake.

To 'up the ante' a bit, chief residents also serve as the manager of hospital interns – they're on call for every question.

A Personal Story: Figure It Out

When I was on call, I had a policy for the interns.

"Figure it out first, unless obviously, it's something crazy or an emergency. Besides, if it's an emergency, the hospital's going to call you on the overhead anyway and tell you that it's code blue or whatever the case may be."

It's 10:30, I'm trying to get some rest upstairs in one of the private staff rooms, and there's a knock at the door before I could even make it to the bed. I swing it open, and there's one of the interns. "Sir, I didn't want to bother you. I know you told me not to call you, but this patient stopped breathing and is not breathing anymore."

A moment of silence... "They're dying."

"Well, that's a good reason to call," I recall answering, and we began heading down to the patient's bed. In retrospect, that intern made the right call; he was in a moment of panic and didn't freeze. Instead of staying still and praying for it to be over, he came and got help. That takes skill and knowledge – knowing when to move and not stand by.

This patient in question had been with us for nearly two months. The family would never come by. They would only call to see if he was alive. He was pretty much brain dead, but he wasn't officially brain dead, just on the cusp. It wasn't a great existence, for sure.

Essentially, he would "code blue" every few days, causing us to rush in and resuscitate him. His family, of course, did not want to exercise a DNR – the refusal to resuscitate. He had no function or quality of life. This time we weren't successful. It wouldn't have mattered if we were there ten minutes earlier; it was his time.

The next day the family came in, upset that he died. It didn't take much investigation to show that his family was cashing in his social security checks – of course, he needed to be alive to continue receiving them.

Doctor 101

Your coat is to your knees; you're on your own. Are you going to be a good or a bad doctor? How do you tell the difference?

The answer is deceptively simple. The bad surgeon doesn't know what to do in the face of adversity or the unexpected. The good surgeon will pull through, just like we've gone through in these examples. They're able to save their patient's life.

A Personal Story: Lab

In my days of being an attending doctor, I found myself down in the catheterization lab on a pretty quiet afternoon. I'm on edge, though, because next door, in the other unit, is a physician that is well-known for having catastrophes – he's performing surgery.

I start hearing shouts.

"Pressure's dropping!"

"Heart rate's dropping!"

Before I know it, the man has gone code blue, and alarms are going off. Hearing the commotion and the alarms blaring in the next lab over, I rushed over, seeing what I was expecting. He has his hands folded, his arms wrapped, and the staff is looking at him for what to do. He doesn't know what to do, though. He can't even open his mouth – he's unable to speak. Feet frozen in place. His staff were the ones calling out.

The staff desperately looked to me, hoping I'd step in – I'd have to scrub in, though - I couldn't start immediately as I had my patient to attend to in the other operating room. The patient's lucky stars were in alignment as that surgeon's partner came into the room and began saving the day. The patient survived the moment and was moved up to the ICU for monitoring – now, instead of one doctor on the case, there were two. Two possible floating ducks. Well-deserved, in this case.

The patient died a day later in the ICU. Two doctors were now open to lawsuits rather than one. The physician had slipped up and opened an artery, effectively giving the patient a heart attack right there on the table.

There's another lesson in this. Even in an emergency situation, you want to slow down. Think about it. Think about the examples that have taken place during your residency, during your training, during your experience in seeing what you've seen, think about what the next step is going to be before you actually make the cut or the decision that could change or end a life.

Alright, we've got the rungs of the ladder to becoming a doctor down, but what about the frame of the ladder itself? Do you understand the systems at work?

INSURANCE 101

Insurance companies are large institutions as well. The factory analogy still applies – customers leave the end of their production chain with policies in hand to use whenever the need arises. In the same way, as with most large hospitals, insurance companies are privately held by corporations and must answer to shareholders in terms of profitability and performance – those statistics have to, without a doubt, stay high. Investors and shareholders demand a return on their investment, or they'll bail, and the company will crumble.

For-profit hospitals: it's in the name. It is their goal to put money in a bank account. These hospitals are also not obligated to provide specific services. This is why you'll find hospitals in geographic areas offer varying specialties of treatment, but most do not cater to all – just as a snow cone shop probably wouldn't open in Antarctica, a hospital won't open a cancer ward in an area that statistically doesn't see many cancer cases.

At the end of it all, it's a numbers game.

Let's make up a common example – sad but true. A customer has a general mid-level policy, makes payments regularly, and has no doctor visits. Twelve good months go by, nothing, then they die in a car accident through no fault of their own.

This is an optimal case for the insurance company, as they were constantly paid by the customer with no payments going out for claims or doctor visits. Insurance isn't a patient-oriented business, it is a finance-oriented business, a cost analysis of who the insured are. All they're doing is evaluating their age, risk factors, and all the other medical issues that are related legal-wise. From the results of the said formula, they're charged, and the company makes a profit.

Barcodes

When a customer calls their insurance company to ask policy questions, the agent on the other end of the line has no idea who they are – they're identified by their policy number. This is why the automated phone system asks them for it ahead of time or looks it up. In yet another parallel, it is the same situation within the walls of a hospital. Reception will create a case number for a patient, and this case number will be scanned at every turn to calculate their bill. This case number will record everything from medications used to treatments ordered.

The 'I-Need-to-Go-to-the-Hospital' Checklist

Prospective patients need to consider the answers to the following questions ahead of time. It could save their lives:

1. "Will my insurance be accepted?"
   Simply enough, does the hospital accept their insurance coverage? Not all hospitals accept every insurance provider point-blank; this is especially true for specialty insurance or policies provided by regional brokers.
2. "What hospital will I need to go to? Can I simply go to the closest one, or do my conditions require special treatment?"
3. "Will the doctors at the hospital I've picked have enough knowledge about my problems to be able to treat me successfully?"
   For example, you wouldn't take an issue surrounding a recent liver transplant to a hospital that has no transplant facilities.

CASH FLOW 101

Given it isn't an extreme case where you aren't bleeding to death or actively in the middle of birthing a baby, you'll go through a process that looks mostly the same at every hospital.

You're taken to the intake desk where all of your insurance information will be recorded, then you'll be given a scannable bracelet – this will be scanned the entire time you're in the building, and it is off to the treatment races from there.

The fun part for the hospital, and the most intense for your wallet, is that the hospital is legally able to, and will, levy fees and upcharges that seemingly make no sense.

A bottle of aspirin may cost $10 down the street at the local pharmacy, but if you're given aspirin from the hospital's pharmacy, that may be $30. This is the same aspirin, just from a stockroom rather than a shelf at the store.

Concerning Money Matters

Here's a dirty secret. Private surgery clinics are held to the very same health and safety laws as full hospitals, and their prices for services are often lower. If you aren't in a case of life-or-death or on Medicare/Medicaid, call around and find a surgery center that offers the surgery you need. Your insurance company will be pleased with the decision as well, as they will not be forced to pay hospital fees.

Medicare and Medicaid Explained

Let's break them down.

Medicare is a government healthcare program for persons aged 65 and up, as well as those with a qualifying disability or medical condition. Medicare Parts A and B are provided by the federal government, but Medicare Parts C and D are provided by private insurance firms and are supervised by the federal government. If a hospital system takes one, it could take some or all.

Medicaid is a state-run program that assists persons with lower or no income and resources with healthcare costs, with different programs available for different demographics. Medicaid plans vary by state, but benefits are consistent across the country.

On the flip side, the business side of the coin, are you happy with seeing older clients with Medicare? You could always decline to take Medicare clients, sticking to private carriers and dictating your own rates. Alternatively, you can still take private carriers, but Medicaid as well, knowing that you'll either be forced to take a set rate or to go into difficult negotiations.

Remember, when you deal with the government, you're dealing with a lot of rules and regulations. They always want a piece of the pie back. They always want to discipline you if you make a minor misstep. They always want a way to get a coupon. It's like any other business.

On a Personal Finance Note

If you are or ever have been employed in a W2 capacity, you've paid out for Medicare and Medicaid as part of your biweekly taxes alongside social security taxes.

If you ever think about what's happening, are you paying for your care? Sure, through your own private insurance, but likely not through Medicare or Medicaid. Essentially, through taxes, you're paying for someone else's insurance, someone you don't even know.

Looking a bit deeper, the system is similar to a Ponzi scheme. A portion is taken from your account and added to the pot to give to everyone else in a trickle-down effect. That's the very definition.

Why is it that we are forced to pay into the pot for everybody else, could there not be a percentage of funds that went straight to the current largest need for the country as a whole? There have been repeated conversations that the Social Security Administration will run dry before the generation currently paying in will be able to reap the benefits.

Think of it this way: if you're earning more than 225,000 a year as a physician, the upper tax bracket, you're paying a tax, the highest tax bracket, which is 42%. You're going to pay for Medicare. You're going to pay for Medicaid. That's quite a chunk of change from each paycheck.

You're paying for social security, none of which you're getting. By the end of the day, when you're done with everything, you're going to keep less than 30% of your earnings. When you've got family and kids to take care of, that doesn't leave a lot of cash in the bank.

In this case, having other sources of income sounds like a great plan, right?

The hospital system has the constant assurance of always being able to accept Medicare and Medicaid. Our practices have the constant assurance of the fact that there will always be clients who need help and private insurers to pay for their care.

However, what's your personal backup assurance?

LEGALESE 101

Of course, we all know the basics; we've all seen the same story on the news or on any medical drama show on Netflix – the patient sues the doctor that botched their surgery, or they sue the doctor falsely in the hopes of a big payday. However, the big question is, how is anyone sure that there really is strength in the case being presented? That's where medical error comes into play.

Defensive Medicine

If you've ever had to go through a medical procedure or the process of diagnosing a medical problem, you'll know this fact well; you'll be put through seemingly test after test, and it begins to feel like some of the tests are just 'for fun' or to pad the bill.

While it is true that patients can be over-tested, there's also a 'method in the madness.' For every test conducted, the doctor and hospital system are adding a layer of protection in the case that there is a lawsuit. There's a term for this concept, 'defensive medicine,' all for the sake of being able to say "Well, we tried every test under the sun to be sure!"

Tort reforms are constantly changing at every level of government, being bounced around more than a volleyball on a hot beach. No matter the geographic location, though, the broad idea still distills into the same essence: each state has begun to put controls on the amount of damages a plaintiff can receive in a case where damages are awarded. As doctors, these changes are helping us a bit, sure, but they aren't comprehensive coverage by any means.

A Personal Story: It Happened to Me

The story starts off inanely, to be quite honest; a case for an abdominal aneurysm repair was referred to my office, as this patient was considered very high risk and had been turned down by a number of other vascular surgeons.

Why was she turned down? The nature of the surgery itself; she was a heavy smoker with lung problems, diabetes, cholesterol out of control, a number of factors all were stewing in her chart. In order for her to have surgery, it looked likely that she would need to be opened abdominally in order to be able to access all problem points. Of course, with the nature of her case, the likelihood there would be complications was through the roof, almost astronomically high.

However, we did receive good news after her first consultation; it was possible that we could do a percutaneous repair, where we would not have to open her chest cavity for access. In fact, it would easily be performed using a stent procedure.

Preparing for the surgery, more tests were performed; it came to light that she'd do better if she was able to have a cardiac bypass surgery ahead of time in order to clear the way for the stent. She saw a specialist and was refused the surgery.

We had no choice but to go in under less-than-optimal conditions, but it was the repair or her life; we knew what we had to do. We simply knew that we had tried to rule out as much of the unknown as possible. It was time for the rubber to meet the road.

Before the aneurysm repair even began, she was complaining of abdominal pain, but there was no time for additional tests. During the aneurysm repair, it was discovered that she had a what's called hematoma growing inside – her blood was pooling outside of the vessels. We did as much as we could, repaired the aneurysm, and left her to recover, with that process taking a few days before she could go home.

It wasn't long after that she went home that it was discovered she had lung cancer; we gave her some better tools to help with the battle, but she died four years later.

Not long after, I received papers from a lawyer, beginning a lawsuit proceeding by her family against myself and my office. Alarmed, my lawyer assured me that it would not hold up well under questioning that the family was pressing a case against the hematoma, a malpractice case when it was four years later that she died; the repair bought her that time, it didn't take it away.

As this was the beginning of COVID, the initial conference between myself, my lawyer, and the family was conducted over video. There was the husband, who I had begun to know well, and his two children, who I'd never seen before.

Her husband's uncomfortable look said it all – he knew the truth. His children were looking for some extra cash. It wasn't about anything else.

My lawyer didn't leave much to the imagination in his opening. "You realize that what Dr. Siddiqui did was surgery on someone who had less than a 2% chance of living. She survived that surgery. He took major risks for doing that. Did you know the risk of dying from COVID and stepping outside of your house is higher than 2%, sir?"

The children didn't say a thing.

Two days later, a call came in, the lawyer informing us that the case was to be dropped. He would be issuing the court paperwork to dismiss the case.

There's a lesson to reiterate here; be honest, be upfront, but be very practical with your patients; it's not about being right or wrong. It's about embracing the truth and reacting properly with the tools you have.

Have you been given a Contract?

Remember something; there are only so many new doctors in training graduating every year, and there is a very high demand for doctors of all types around the United States. When someone hands you a contract to look at, you better have a lawyer look at it, and you better ask for more than what they're giving you – they can afford it, and they need you.

Your goal is to make the most, as much as you can. No compromising just because you've been in their hamster wheel at one point. You're a free hamster out to battle your own way in order not to be a hamster anymore. You know that you're doing and what's best for you.

The hospital system and insurance companies aren't there to help you, their goal is to get you as cheap labor, and you're a pawn. Their shareholders can't do the surgeries themselves and wouldn't want to anyway. Even when negotiating your contract, you become your own business. You make your own rules. When they offer you $400,000, ask them for $600,000 and see what they say.

The worst thing they're going to say is, "No, but let's see if we can meet in the middle." You could easily get yourself some vacation days or bonus potential; if not, more money goes directly into your pocket. Just because it is given to you does not mean that it is set in stone.

Inevitabilities

It doesn't matter how good a doctor you are, whether you're the best surgeon you can be or the worst. You're still going to get sued. Every physician in seven to ten years is going to have at least one lawsuit. Remember, lawsuits aren't automatically judge and jury – many are frivolous, or outright attempts at fraud, in hopes that the charged emotions of a death or medical scenario will drum up either sympathy from the judge or a quick settlement to keep it quiet. Settlements are the name of the game. The patient makes money, and everybody walks. Don't forget the whole 'unsaid' visual of a settlement, though.

"They paid to get it over with and have nothing else said."

That's an open-ended statement with no real answer, for better or worse.

Lobbyists: Devil's Advocates?

In government, you've got plenty of lobbyists sitting there trying to get rules and regulations passed. They spend all day, every day, chasing after the representatives that can be potentially swayed into helping get their agenda passed.

'Big Pharma' is one of the biggest, nastiest, smartest lobbying groups out there. Their goal is to get certain drugs, medications, vaccines, and laws passed in a way to increase profits. Think of 'Big Pharma' lobbyists as drug sales reps on steroids.

The FDA

Let's say the FDA approves a pacemaker or defibrillator from a big company, and two years later, the very same device is recalled. Not a good look, right?

The FDA decides to recall the device; you see this all the time, whether it's in the news or everywhere else – they recall this pacemaker or defibrillator for constant issues. Smart, predatory lawyers out there are keeping an eye on this.

The bad news is, if you're one of the doctors who used the equipment, you'll likely be getting a letter. These lawyers climb the entire ladder, suing the device company, the rep, health systems, and doctors who used the product. If you're an independent doctor, this is where you get the short end of the stick.

The device company will protect itself and its reps. The health system will defend itself and its employees.

Who will protect you?

Drug Reps: The Real Wolves in Sheep Suits

As for the drug and machine reps, rolling back to them, they're going to wine and dine you. They earned themselves a bachelor's in biology. Maybe they plan to even go on to medical school, but now they're working as drug reps – they're attractive young ladies or attractive young men.

They take you out to dinners. They take you on ski trips and pay your entire way to attend conferences around the globe. Plus, as they're looking to sell you on a big contract, they'll sweet-talk you all day. At the end of the day, it is the rep's job to attract you to them long enough to get you to sign on the dotted line. You can imagine what can take place when you're going on trips together. It's almost like going on really great dates – they're interested in you; they're paying for everything.

Interestingly, most states have created kickback laws, seeing to it that doctors receive only a certain amount of money for their kickbacks, not huge paychecks that can open up the doorways to luxury cars and new houses. Very interestingly enough, the same has not been done with congressmen or senators, though they affect lives just as much through laws and policy.

Here's a tip to avoid a bad decision – make them meet your office manager.

Your office manager will be your shield. Unless the drug rep presents a real case with statistics and proof, they'll be out on the street in a snap. Otherwise, you will be inundated with drug reps in your office every day and night throughout all days and hours. You'll be spending not only your business day, but also after-hours at endless dinners. With the office manager, not a chance!

Should the rep get through the first hurdle, the next stage is they'll be going on a tour with you – from there, you can start the decision process on whether to sign a deal or not.

Secondly, before anything is signed, you need to do research on your own. You are educated enough. Put all of that schooling to good use. Remember, you'll be on the line to prescribe 'this' pill or use 'that' machinery. Is it going to improve your practice or hinder you?

Why not make the best decision and use the best medication out there for your patient? Always choose what's best for your patient. Not for you. Whatever you do, it is going to affect you. Later down the road, they now publish and print information on how much each doctor was paid by whatever company that they were a speaker for, or getting kickbacks from, for example.

Sure, you may receive a few hundred grand in speaking fees; however, your patients are going to read about what you're doing. It's public; they will know everything. That few hundred in speaking fees will be spent quickly if your practice begins to dwindle.

Nothing is free in this life.

CHAPTER 7

GOING OFF-ROAD

In March of 2019, I cashed out my hard work by selling off my clinic and transitioning into the hospital system, still doing work on the clinician side, just not on the same level as owning and operating the full clinic on my own. It was a downsizing move to accommodate my family and personal goals, giving me more free time to concentrate on them.

As the COVID pandemic geared into its first wave, most physicians blew it off as another virus, attributing the craze to the media and social media hype going around. Most of us in the medical community continued along as is, simply adjusting as mandates came around, sometimes with an eye roll. I was busy settling back into a hospital system; sure, I was staying up on current news, but I was busy; it wasn't a prime concern in my mind.

By early summer, I came to realize my own hubris around the situation – it finally came home to nest that the situation was no joke. Despite my fears, I continued on. Again, business as usual, even though, by this point, I was making sure that my staff and I were taking precautions.

In June of 2020, I was exposed to the virus – a few COVID-positive attendees, even though they were unaware, came into close contact with me. I learned the news a few days later, as a few of those COVID-positive people now had fully developed symptoms.

I'll be honest with the fact that I was terrified; I've had a history of underlying asthma – of course, the medical literature I'd been reading up until that point (and still through today) made a point of expressing the fact that COVID patients with underlying conditions, especially those dealing with the pulmonary system, were in particular danger.

Wouldn't you know, before June was over, I was sick. Three to four weeks of it. All the while, I knew what danger I was in – even with the few studies available at the time, the writing was on the wall. I'd been seeing it and dealing with it but being sick with it was a whole new ballgame – one where I had little equipment other than the smarts in my head.

At first, I was home-bound, recovering on my own. Predictably, though, with the symptoms not fully clearing away, it took a short hospital stay to finish kicking the virus out. I was talking steroid and IV treatments from a hospital bed. Sitting in the hospital bed, glad I wasn't in a state where I needed to be put on a ventilator, I was given plenty of time to think.

My entire outlook on life changed. "I want to enjoy every moment, I don't know what's going to happen tomorrow, and to some extent, I can't predict it. I'm young, punches are going to come my way. I just have to accept that fact."

Of course, the treatments did help, and I was released from the hospital shortly after. While I felt okay, I wasn't truly up to the challenge of returning to work yet, so I took the time to travel a bit, Colorado to ski and hike, then on to Peru to visit Machu Picchu. Sounds like a great time, right? Altitude sickness had never bothered me before, there were no red flags as to reasons why we should delay the trip.

Well, there were complications. Altitude sickness struck, spurred on by my underlying asthma and complications from the ongoing COVID, which, as we know, lingers for quite a while in terms of long-term side effects. I knew I was in trouble when we arrived in Cusco. That's the closest city to the Machu Picchu site, around 13,000 miles above sea level.

I woke up the first night there, at three in the morning, unable to take a single breath. The moment I sat up, startling my wife awake, I found myself opening my mouth, blood-tinged frothy sputum falling out onto my hands and the blankets. From what you likely inferenced, you're right – I was spitting up blood, a common sign of a disease called Pulmonary Edema.

From my bedroom, feeling worse than before, I couldn't help but spend more time thinking about what got me to take those trips in the first place, that initial revelation. I couldn't help but remember and was thankful that I did my estate planning sessions years earlier, as well as the endless meetings with attorneys, balance sheets, and will proofreading. It was a mental triathlon, not to mention expensive to carry out.

"I'm going to live my life no longer fearing tomorrow. I'm going to live for today. If I'm comfortable and happy, I'm going to travel; I'm going to live how I'd like. If I want to work past 65, I will; if I want to stop and travel, I will. I'm not going to let some societal idea change what I do."

But first, I had to get out of there. My wife continually begged me to hold back my coughs, fearing they'd believe that I had COVID, and we would be put under a secondary quarantine. I then used my skills of knowledge, training my entire life in medicine. I asked my wife to call the front desk. We were in luck, they had oxygen and tubes ready, as tourists suffering from altitude sickness isn't uncommon. I was hooked up, plus with an oxygen meter which wasted no time in announcing my Oxygen level of 70, extremely low. I sit back, relax, and bring my level back up to

90, knowing that I'd just dodged a bullet – anything below 70 and you're automatically carted off to the hospital.

We had a flight to catch that afternoon. Problem being, I cannot bring the oxygen on the plane. It's clear, to survive the flight, the multiple depressurizations, will I need some steroids, IV steroids, plus something called Lasix, which is a water pill?

Of course, we're in a foreign country where everyone speaks Spanish, and we're two plain-faced English speakers. I look at my wife, Natalie, showing her a picture of IV Lasix on my phone. She takes the phone, photo plastered on the screen, knowing her mission. She had to get the medicine on her own, there'd be no telling the hotel, they'd have us shipped off to the hospital.

A half a mile block, walking, and she manages to find a building that is pretty obviously a pharmacy. She makes her way in, trying to look inauspicious, and gets the attention of the pharmacist, showing the picture on the screen of my cell phone. She's pointing, gesturing, unable to speak a word of usable Spanish outside of "Hola."

After some animated convincing and flashing of my hospital badge, Natalie manages to get the medicine and bring it back.

I'm concerned when she walks in; she looks happy, but a little dejected. "They had what you wanted, but no inhalers." I breathe deeply, knowing that it's going to be a little more difficult now, but still doable.

Looking over the medicines, I hold my hand out for the needles – she plops one large needle onto the palm of my hand. I keep holding it out, expecting the other, smaller needle – the one that is used to inject the medication – the one she's handed me is the one used to extract and prep the medication into an IV bag.

Nothing.

"That's all she gave me." Natalie said, turning pale.

That needle had to have been the size of a pen. Usually, we use one large needle to extract the liquid and the smaller one to inject into the patient.

"Oh, well, I've got to inject myself."

As difficult as it is to do, I roll myself onto my stomach, draw up the fluid, and stab myself – yes, in the butt, injecting the medicine as far as I could before Natalie had to step in, hands shaking, to finish the injection.

After an hour, I feel okay, and we make it to the airport in time, even if Natalie is still shaken up. The air pressure in the cabin helps me to get some extra air into my lungs – by the time we land again on native soil, my oxygen is in the nineties, perfectly safe territory.

Six months later my wife and I were with another physician and his wife, having dinner, and we tell this story, getting a laugh out of it. However, we're 'dead-seriously' stopped at the 'stop coughing' part. The other physician couldn't help but look over at Natalie. "Do you know, the mortality rate is over 50% with what he had?" She had no clue, but I didn't expect her to know. I knew and didn't say anything, but I also knew if I panicked, she would have handled it differently.

LOOKING BACK ON HISTORY

In fact, we are much weaker than these viral organisms causing every deadly outbreak through human history (e.g., the medieval plague, or the Spanish Flu of the early 1900s). No matter the setting, these tiny little creatures with little to no brains can completely pull humanity down as a whole to a basic level. That's what you call the 'ultimate reality check.'

Much like in our own image as humans, these viruses and bacteria are able to mutate; they're able to change. They're able to adjust their ways to come back and fight as science strikes back. It truly is a constant back-and-forth effort. One lays out a blow, the other backs up and packs its punch. Repeat, rinse, and repeat.

We've got great pharmaceutical companies staffed with the best scientists out there that are coming in with vaccines and treatments. That's true, however, at the same time, they are in the business to make money. Pharmaceutical companies aren't nonprofits – they're out to make money from their treatments to patent their research and charge a premium to use it.

In another five to ten years, there will be another outbreak of some scary new virus. Bird flu, swine flu, Ebola, COVID, what's next? We are unable to defeat any viruses in totality; all of these will still be out there in twenty years, just as polio technically still exists. The fact is that they'll simply dissolve into the background and become less important as we build our security systems to detect and defend against them. Science has changed at a pace unknown in human history within the past one hundred years; we've gone from horses and buggies to atomic bombs and cars that can drive themselves. There's a certain element of peace in that fact.

Progress Makes Us Human

This chapter could seem like it's all doom and gloom, but in all reality, it isn't. It's a hopeful one. The bright spot, this example being COVID, is that eventually, as the human species, we'll overcome. We're able to do things on a much faster timeline when under pressure, both on our own as individuals and as a species, which was great for our country in terms of fighting COVID. However, what's more interesting is that the virus doesn't have any clue about this. In essence, we're able to pack three punches as compared to the virus' one.

In the case of COVID, one year later, after the original strain, it changed to a Delta, a modified variant. That's a quick mutation, less than a year. From there, it will mutate again, and it will continuously mutate. It's here to stay, the virus is smart.

This is where staying ahead is essential, and the great news is that we're doing just that. Eventually, we're going to gain a spot on the curve just as we have for the flu and polio. We'll be able to swat away mutations as they come – we'll be the king of the hill.

And as a result, when enough versions of the COVID vaccine roll out, they will not be optimally effective, as no vaccine for routine illnesses like the flu are, but they'll put up a significant barrier. Anyone who contracts COVID who has had their vaccine may still get sick. However, the symptoms will go from hospitalization level to simply staying home and having soup for a few days. We're not there yet, but that's what the goal is, and the scientific community agrees that as long as we keep fighting, we'll be there sooner rather than later. The line is being drawn in the sand, and we're getting there, fighting against each wave from the ocean of uncertainty that threatens to erase it.

STAYING AHEAD

When you look at the big picture, not just in medicine, but at the big picture of life, the goal is to know where you're going. We all fear the unknown and do our best to stay ahead of it, even if that effort is purely on our subconscious, which it is most of the time.

- What are my goals right now?
- What are my goals three to five years from now?
- What do I ultimately want to do?

These are the questions that consistently run through the back of our mind, as if on tape.

You know, it's a common question in an interview situation. "Where do you see yourself five years and ten years from now?"

While the question comes loaded with good intentions, I don't think people really sit down and think about the question. They just spit something out that sounds good at that moment.

Although it sounds cliché, it is true that part of life is simply staying ahead of that routine question. "What are you going to be doing in X years?"

Have your list ready, know where you're going. Just like you'd never go on an expedition to climb Mount Everest without a plan, you can't embark on a mission to take control of your life and succeed without a game plan, either.

WHAT UNPREDICTABILITY SAYS ABOUT THE MEDICAL SYSTEM

Part of being human is that we, of course, make mistakes. As doctors, sometimes we lose that human instinct where we care about others, or we imagine others in our own positions or not as patients. It's easy to pass off patients who lash out in the moment as just someone who is rude in general, not someone who has been simmering under the pressure cap of stress and pain for weeks or months. We almost imagine them as if there are no emotions inside of their head or even our own, then the emotions start to go away, leaving only charts and numbers behind.

That's where we begin to enter dangerous territory. As a doctor, you begin growing apathetic, and the patient becomes a number in the same way as an insurance company or hospital looks at them. Literally, we start to see them as a cog in the machinery rather than as a human being with feelings.

As physicians, we're covered up with our masks, gloves, gowns, shoe covers, and all the typical equipment as part of protocol. It's a scary image, even for a patient who has been through the process hundreds of times. Remember, we all have a deep-seated fear of death somewhere in our minds. It is as programmed into us as our fight-or-flight instinct.

As medical providers, we need to understand that everything happening around us affects our patients, mentally and emotionally. Our patients live in a world of 'I don't know' – that's practically the underlying definition of 'diagnosis' – an exploratory process to discover the cause of an illness. Every day is a new discovery, and sometimes, those discoveries are life-changing for the worse.

The business and bureaucracy of the hospital system are elements we all have to deal with – both as providers and patients – they're like vacuums that can easily suck the humanity out of the process. The systems are built in a way that, emotionally, never helps. While some of those rules are for the better, such as not allowing extra close contact outside of what is necessary due to COVID protocols, we also have to recognize that there is always an element of bad mixed in with the good – less personal contact means no opportunity to hug a patient or put a hand on their shoulder.

Let's be honest, all of these things affect you. All of these additional elements make things difficult as a physician to navigate through the waters of professional and private life, to figure out what is the best thing to do. It's easy to get lost in the mist.

However, at the end of the day, you have to see the patient's emotional side and make the best decision for them based on your being in that situation. You should never put a patient into a situation that you yourself wouldn't want, or couldn't bear, to be in.

There's a theme here. It's our duty to look at both sides – both as the provider and the patient.

Looking at things from the other perspective, I think we can open our minds, stay flexible, and strive to be more empathetic human beings all around. When faced with the unimaginable, it's important to go in swinging. That's critical. However, it is just as important to be prepared ahead of time.

CHAPTER 8

THE FUTURE OF MEDICINE

Technology isn't going anywhere. It's here to stay, and we have to learn how to live alongside it, to make it work for us, and to prevent technology from becoming a crutch – this is an uphill battle because we already know that it is an addiction in many of our lives.

There's the first hurdle to overcome, and in the world of facial recognition, license plate scanning, social credit, and deepfakes, it seems as if I could be misleading. There is no universal storage of medical files.

Portable Lifestyles

Take the 'snowbirds,' for example, everyone's elderly aunts, uncles, grandmas, and grandpas that make the trip south every winter to escape the harsh winters at their homes up north, be it at a condo, apartment, RV park, or seaside shack. From Canada to Michigan, cars and planes are packed to capacity to make their way to Florida and other sunny states every year.

In my own case, when these snowbirds come down to see us in Florida for about six to eight months a year, as they aren't taking a vacation from their health responsibilities, then, just as they came, they leave, heading back up north, leaving us at some stage in the treatment process to be resumed with their other doctor 'back home.'

For example, let's say a patient had a full CT back home before coming south to my clinic in Florida. If this is the case, we have to request their records, call their doctor back home, and request that their records be transferred. This takes time, wasted time. It would be much easier if there was a national way of looking up their medical records and seeing what had already been done, almost like a Facebook of medical information – a great library of our patients' histories – to pull from quickly and effectively.

Well, then there's the other choice of trying to find documents, making mistakes, costing both time and money. All of this is well known, and we still operate somewhat in the land of the dinosaurs – documents have to be signed for, then faxed over digitally. Read that line again – faxed. Most of us don't even remember how to use a fax machine.

Take a note here.

Everyone should carry their own medical records, whether they're snowbirds or college-age. We live in a world of digital copies. There's no excuse. I still see this to this day. We carry our cell phones with us everywhere, why not have a PDF copy of your most important records ready to go? If you're in a catastrophic car accident, for example, precious hours could be lost trying to fetch your medical history, hours that would be better spent treating your wounds.

KNOW YOUR OPTIONS

You have two options when it comes to having surgery. You can have it at the hospital or a surgery center, an outpatient setting, or the third option for general health, adding in urgent cares as well.

If you need to see a doctor and it's not urgent, you need to go to an office visit – you've done it yourself for those ingrown toenails, bothersome sore throats, and sprained fingers. These are the minor annoyances in life that we can live with until our

GP has time to see us. If your usual GP isn't open or doesn't have any times that work available, this would be the moment to visit an urgent care, simply making sure that you keep any medical paperwork you're given, and that you relay what happened to your GP.

However, if you need to have a hernia repaired or open-heart surgery stemming from a heart attack, for example, it often isn't a matter of waiting until a hand-selected surgeon has an opening. If the condition has progressed far enough, it's about who will save your quality of life, if not your entire life. They've got the ICU beds to save you, the emergency medical equipment, and the surgeons on staff to carry the operation through.

If not one of these extreme cases, for anything else under the sun, you need to go to a surgery center, not wait to be sent to an emergency department – always.

First, you've got a higher risk of infections being in the emergency room – you know this and have likely just never thought about it. Imagine the emergency room. When you go there, you've got the concept of being in rooms or being on a floor with other sick patients, sure, but just how dangerous is this setting?

Think of it. You have the waiting room where all patients, no matter what condition, are lumped together. You've got the hacking and coughing possible infectious flu patient sitting beside the gunshot victim, next to the person with a cut finger dripping fluid, next to the hypochondriac just waiting for a reason to be seen. Even after that, the extent of your 'room' will likely be a bed separated by a curtain.

Surgery centers are always the preferable option. You would be treated better, work with a surgeon you know, and receive the same quality of treatment as if you were in the largest hospital system. Surgery centers are a clear winner in this boxing match.

At first, it is true, the number of services these centers could perform was a niche list; however, as gains have been made against the lobbyists of hospital systems, the list has opened up to generally any option and elective surgery under the sun.

GOING VIRTUAL

As with culture and education, we're moving into a world of more and more technology—in our case, virtual medicine. As an example, the now-classic one, COVID – it has turned the medical world upside down, making everything short of surgery into telemedicine.

Let's face it, telemedicine is going to stick around now that it has started, and the kinks have been forcibly worked out. Hospital systems no longer have to worry about sanitizing crowded waiting rooms, working around possible HIPAA violations through wandering patients or wandering eyes, dealing with parking, and handling the salaries of many maintenance men and cleaners to keep the facility clean due to the high rates of in-and-out traffic. Doctors themselves love telemedicine, as they often can conduct their meetings from the privacy and comfort of their home offices. They never even have to go in for at least a few days of the week as they meet with patients to discuss cases.

The patient interaction factor has been halved. Sure, that can be a positive. However, as we've touched on before, this 'soullessness' can lead us down a scary path of 'medicine run by robots.' There's no humanity to be found in cold silicone screens, no matter how much we love our computers and cell phones for their easy access to TikTok, Instagram, and Candy Crush.

Soulless Medicine

The patient turns off their screen, sometimes in tears or emotionally exhausted from having received bad news, and the connection is over – literally and emotionally. In offices, we're able to stand, put a hand on their shoulder, and look into their eyes, to step in and briefly hide the lab coat to do what any human would do. Over cell phones, we're just the end of a dead connection, a black Zoom call window.

In the world of telemedicine, we go from being 'my doctor' to being 'a doctor,' a face on a screen who delivers bad news without care, ready to charge a credit card or insurance account.

Strangely enough, we're quickly approaching an era where that face on the other side might not even be a real doctor, but an AI piece of software designed to look and sound like a doctor, simply using a searchable database and live interfacing to do the same thing a real-life human doctor would. The problem is, how do you bring up problems with an AI-generated lifeform? If worst comes to worst, how do you sue one?

The World of Holistic Care

Holistic has a simple definition – to handle the sum of all parts. The big idea of holistic healthcare is that patients are more than just their targeted conditions – they must have their emotions, self-care, and other physical problems managed at the same time to achieve recovery and full health.

Holistic healthcare obviously isn't the modus operandi of the modern privatized healthcare system of 'charge 'em and get 'em out.'

Misleading Misnomers

Many physicians calling themselves 'holistic practitioners' are unintentionally lying to their patients – what they're truly practicing is a meld of preventative medicine with concierge medicine.

For example, stress tests (running on a treadmill), active monitoring, and electrocardiograms are the most common ways that doctors can scan for heart disease. However, getting signed up for one of these tests can be a minefield of hurdles.

Heart disease is one of the number one killers in the American population – it's higher than breast cancer. It's higher than most cancers combined, yet there are no set guidelines to map out the most common risk factors and how to catch them. When the disease is already there, it's too late. If you've got a family history of diabetes, high cholesterol, you're overweight, you've got sleep apnea, then the warning signs are there.

Why is it that you have to have complaints to be treated or even examined? Often, by the time enough symptoms pile up to mandate a test, damage has already been done. The hospital, insurance, and governmental policy systems at work in the United States are currently dictating when or when you cannot have a stress test, electrocardiogram, or active monitoring for a set period, performed. What would happen if a patient had the power to order one up as easily as they can order up a cheeseburger at a drive-up window? Within the current climate, if a patient isn't showing signs of chest pain, they are not going to get approved for a stress test.

Essentially, COVID has changed the mindset of individuals saying, 'we want to live longer.' Sure, patients can technically order up any test; they'll just be forced to pay for it 'out of pocket' rather than by insurance. However, these cases are becoming increasingly true, where patients take on tests and scans to simply improve their overall health or to prove to themselves that they are healthy. Holistic care, in that aspect, that example, is real.

If I want to get a CT scan to make sure I don't have any brain cancer, I should be able to. If I want to check the arteries in my neck and my legs for blockages, sure, I should be able to get one.

As a real-life example, look at the age of colonoscopy patients – they're growing younger and younger. Look at Chadwick

Boseman, the actor in *Black Panther*, who died at a very young age of colorectal cancer – a death completely preventable, would it have been caught by a colonoscopy and treated.

Preventative and holistic healthcare options are going to grow in popularity to the point that the systems in place that once repressed them will have to begin taking them seriously. They'll have to adapt, to find ways to have those styles make financial sense for their business models, whether they like it or not.

MEDICINE OF THE FUTURE

Obviously, millennial doctors are going to lean towards telehealth over face-to-face interaction. After all, they will have trained up through the COVID period – it'll be what's familiar, paired with our own personal lifestyles of being device-addicted. Feels natural, right?

As the baby boomer generation cycles out, replaced with more tech-savvy Generation X'ers, telehealth as a standard will creep further and further into everyday practice, even if telehealth itself hasn't improved outcomes or any single standard of care. It's a fact that there hasn't been enough time for researchers to study the full effects of telehealth on the medical system, as true telehealth options have only existed for around five years.

Where there are bumps in the information superhighway, there are also a few smooth cruising spots. Pharmacies and device providers have developed their own patient-facing apps to improve delivery and help cut back on the chance of missing a refill, for example. In this case, smartphones and telehealth have actually improved access to effective medicine.

Think I'm overexaggerating the mixed bag of effects telehealth has? Think of the last time you had a common cold. You had a fever for a few nights, were sneezing like crazy, felt a little nauseous, tired, and like you could just explode with nasty snot. What did you do, other than lay in bed? Most likely, hop on a symptom checker, plug in everything, then receive a list of possible maladies. Of course, the true diagnosis was likely among the top five possibilities; however, going further down the list, possible diagnoses only became scarier and scarier, not to mention further from the truth. You started with a common cold and ended with brain cancer. Your runny nose was no longer a runny nose, but brain fluid seeping out.

I can't tell you the number of times that I've had a patient call, nearly demanding a certain medication, seemingly for no reason. After being questioned, they reveal their cards, saying that they were searching the internet and found 'Medicine X' that they believe could treat them more efficiently, effectively, and for a lower cost. It's safe to say that they're rarely correct.

Robots and Margins of Error

Robots are starting to take the place of humans in some surgery scenarios. Sure, potential mistakes drop away with the mechanical aspect of robot-assisted surgery, but the time to conduct a surgery goes up, as you're dealing with a machine running mathematical algorithms and following a programmed pattern, unable to adapt on the fly.

The thing is that most insurance companies require a human behind the controls in order to utilize the machinery fully – the human element is never fully removed. I do not think that it will ever completely disappear in these cases.

As a human, the ability to 'turn on a dime' when you're thinking, changes things. Essentially, this ability to think freely is what makes us human. Remember, robots have no feelings. They may have their own versions of 'thoughts,' but they surely don't feel true happiness, sadness, or remorse. They may be able to emulate emotions as part of their programming. Think of *The Sims* if

4

444

you're a fan of video games, but the mechanical being you're looking at isn't truly smiling – a line of code is telling it to do so.

Great surgeons all understand that their patients are just that – patients, not slabs of meat to be experimented on for a paycheck. They have fears. They cry, they feel pain. Robotic surgeries were a topic of curiosity on the original television run of Star Trek twenty years ago. Most upcoming physicians were born at the time that the idea of a patient being sutured by a robotic arm operated by a computer was a pipe dream, something to marvel at on the big screen.

The fact is, we aren't prepared for robot-assisted surgeries. We've never been prepared. We weren't prepared to utilize nuclear power – think of Chernobyl and Three-Mile Island. We weren't quite ready yet to use steam-powered equipment at the turn of the industrial revolution – the first trains often exploded and maimed riders. We definitely weren't ready for the first weapons of war made during the caveman days.

Big Box

When we aren't talking about surgery, we're talking about the other most important aspect, pharmacy. New players in this game are going to be the Walmarts, the Amazons, the Sam's Clubs, and Targets. The big corporations that power our spending habits worldwide.

These multinational conglomerates going into the health business for themselves, is going to be extremely common, with telemedicine becoming the norm. There are large companies right now that are going public on the stock market, the NASDAQ, that are large tele-health corporations, Tele-Doc, for example, is a large tele-health company embraced by many companies as part of their health plans. Why? Because it's cheap to provide.

We're Still Battling Unknowns

Looking through history, we've had issues with viral flus. Swine flu, bird flu, Ebola, and these new viral advancements aren't going to stop, ever. Why isn't there anything being done in that aspect? Why isn't there anything being done to put a stop to it? The answer is easy. The future of medicine is still a concept that no one scientist, not even groups of them, are sure where it will go.

Some say the future isn't in preventative care, as medical problems will arise even in the healthiest of patients. Some scientists say we need to concentrate on medicine, technologies, and techniques to tackle problems as they happen, not to preemptively try and stop them. From there, politics then gets involved. Budgets come up. Ideologies begin to appear and insert themselves, and the crystal ball gets only cloudier. Think it's cloudy enough yet? The last part of the puzzle, big pharma, turns the ball from murky seawater to completely clouded over.

It is true that these systems have their own arm of Medicare and Medicaid right now to charge, as the baby boomer population is still large. However, what happens when this base dries up? Do they extend it out to a lower age range, a younger generation? Those who aren't currently applicable? Young professionals? Young families with jobs, working parents? This will likely be the case, as the cash has to come from somewhere.

Medicare and Medicaid are two organizations too large to be allowed to collapse. They're simply too deeply entrenched in the United States' hospital systems and political culture.

CHAPTER 9

DIFFERENT ROADS, DIFFERENT FUTURES

You've got a conundrum on your hands. There are unlimited possibilities with unlimited doors to go through, it's true. Now isn't the time to freeze, though. If the idea of all these possibilities fills you to the brim with anxiety, know that you've already narrowed some of your path – you chose medicine. With your residency and your internship, you stay the course, narrowing the possibilities a little further.

You get that degree in hand. You can become the hundred-percent hospital doctor, staying on the hospital payroll once you earn your white coat. On the other hand, you can break and become a private practice doctor, which we've already explored at length.

If none of those options sound particularly fulfilling, there are more to consider. What about becoming a doctor for a large pharma company, overseeing trials? What about a scientist developing drugs and treatments? These are options rarely discussed in medical school, but exist, nonetheless.

No matter your path, you can find a way to get a return on your investment.

OVER THE LONG HAUL

At this point, you've spent around eight years in the "learning system" – undergraduate, graduate, internship, and residency. Compare that time commitment to other professionals such as architects, engineers, and other four-year degree-holders who enter the market with six-figure salaries. You're up against a tall order. There's some catching up to do.

Your initial return on investment will be in gratitude. Gratitude for getting where you are and anyone who helped you get there. Those feelings will come crashing over your body somewhere in your first days – be it as an intern, resident, or doctor. However, if your return on investment is looking strictly from a financial stamp point of view, then you'll be facing an upward battle from now until around the halfway mark of your professional life. That's quite a long-haul ride, thinking of your student loans.

Take your take-home income, take out your everyday expenses, your debts – we've all got them. That leaves some funds to help pay off your debts, sure, but there's no treasure trove to pull from. There's a way to speed the process up, though. As Warren Buffet says, the biggest step toward wealth is a diverse portfolio – and he's right.

EXPANDING YOUR FINANCIAL HORIZONS

This can sound like a bunch of real estate or tycoon mumbo-jumbo, but the advice is simple and solid. You need to have multiple sources of income, whether it's in real estate, the stock market, cryptocurrency, having a brokerage account, or even selling medical supplies.

The First Route: Invest!

Of course, doctors and students know medical companies well.

They're always coming in and out pitching new products, showing off new equipment, and generally "wining and dining" anyone they can get to listen. If there's a company you like and believe in, why not invest in them through stocks? After all, by using their products or taking on some of their equipment, aren't you investing in your own success?

Real Estate

Of course, as we've already explored, why not open your own brokerage, and pay rent to yourself rather than a landlord? Given you have extra space in your building, why not rent it out? There are plenty of doctors who can't afford to or don't want to own their own building. They rent their space from you, you build it out to suit, and sit back as the profits roll in each month.

Ready to get out of business or not bother with owning your building anymore? Excellent cap rates are on the market for sellers; it's a win-win scenario.

UNCOMMON ROUTES

Still unsure? Slow down and take a look around. You'll find spaces where a potential business could spring up, even in the unlikeliest of places.

Ever noticed other students in university or medical school struggling to take notes during the lecture?

There's an entire business there. Take the notes during class and resell those notes to other students later down the line in order to prep for exams. Remember, they're stressed, missed class, or simply aren't great note-takers. Other students will pay a premium to make up for their own lack of preparation and still pass upcoming exams.

What sweetens the pot is that by the end of medical school, a note-taker could practically publish a book that could be passed down through the years. Talk about passive income!

Think of every mom on your street or old friends from high school on Facebook, selling aromatherapy products and leggings – that's a diverse portfolio. Maybe not with MLM products, but you can do it too. Speed up your own wealth-building process. Get out there and create!

Seeing Futures

When you're in residency training, you have no idea what's going on in the world. Your life has become an isolated island of work – and you're running on a hamster wheel to keep the waters from sweeping you away. There's a bright spot, though. The end of the tunnel seems just so close by, like the glow of a ship on the horizon of the water around you. Sure, depending on your current point on the timeline, you may need to pick a specialization or move to accommodate finding a better position, which will weigh down that hamster wheel a bit, but you'll still make it through.

Choose Your Own Adventure

This is your own adventure, and you can plot your course. Sure, there's a lot of running on that 'hamster wheel' – however, at some point along the line, you'll be given the steering wheel to your ship. In little bits at first, but later on, to plot full courses for places unknown.

What makes you happy? What do you like to do? Where do you want to be next year, in ten years? Make a choice to actively choose now, not later; the further down the line you "ride things out," letting fate make choices for you, the harder it is to take control and steer things in the way you choose.

Before you know it, you're part of the assembly line, no choices given, simply riding the conveyor belt, letting what will happen, happen. Where's the happiness in that?

Don't do what you're told to do. Do what your heart and mind tell you to do.

CHAPTER 10

FROM SCHOOL TO HOSPITAL

College: Ramen, classes, studying...

Medical school: More ramen, more classes, more studying...

The hospital: Lives and careers on the line, and more ramen...

You're being flushed through the pipeline. Are you going to clog up or make your way through and out into the great beyond? This is your moment of greatest transformation. Take hold of the moment by the horns!

Clinically, you'll be applying everything you've learned the past twenty-five odd years, especially the last eight you've spent in school. It's a surreal, heady transition, like being in a twilight zone episode. One day you're studying in your dorm room, and the next, you're running after a stretcher, code alarm being called out overhead, preparing to save the life of someone you've never met.

It's not a job; it's a life.

THE BIG IDEA: LEARN HOW IT ALL WORKS

In the medical business, we have to be good at math. Here's an equation to break down.

Curiosity + Investigation + Action = Success

Once you master this equation, your entire business format and understanding of your career will begin to change.

Curiosity

Curiosity is a mix of two tenacious factors: self-drive and a big '?' question mark.

If you're one of those individuals that loves to just go to work nine to five and go home for dinner, a drink, and what's on TV, this part of the equation isn't for you.

Investigation

The unknown is out there, waiting to be discovered. Some days, it will come to you, like a patient coming in through the emergency room with a case you've never seen before, and sometimes you'll go to it, wanting to discover or learn something new. Either way, investigation comes into your life; it brings new chances to fly or flop. Which will it be?

Action

It's true, things won't always go your way, but each path is one paved with lessons – you'll come out the other side all the better for the journey.

Success

What can and what won't go wrong? As you know, just about anything in life can take a turn for the worse. We can do something as simple as going to the Starbucks for a cup of coffee and end up scraping our car door on a fire hydrant, perhaps slip and fall getting out of the shower, or get to work five minutes late due to traffic and miss a meeting.

Rehearse your reactions, read, learn, and invest. But most importantly, expect the worst and turn it into an outcome better than if it would have been handed to you. The real definition of 'success' is 'constantly thinking on your feet.' Lives in the medical world are always on the line. The difference between life and death is your reaction – do you freeze or excel?

Different Paths in a Forest Without Trees

Every nurse, nurse practitioner, and, of course, doctor out there, has a specific set of tasks to accomplish that will never change; however, there are more options in life than those that are pre-prescribed:

- Maybe you could simply be a physician within a hospital system your entire life.
- Maybe you could start in a hospital system but expand into your own clinic.
- Maybe you could expand from being a family physician to specializing in bariatric surgery or becoming a psychiatrist.

All of these examples are perfectly fine; they're great ways to achieve a fulfilling career, a comfortable lifestyle, and leading a life worth writing a book about. However, there's also the opportunity to engage in real estate, for example – buying a space to open your own clinic or renting it out to other doctors.

Maybe on top of this, you'd want to distribute medical supplies as a supplier? There's the opportunity to purchase investment stakes and stocks in pharmaceutical companies and device manufacturers that come into your office each day. Maybe you're looking to go a bit further? There are always related industries that are always in demand – think ambulance services, clinic setup consultation, HIPAA security, and many other niches in the medical business that are constantly crying out for hands on deck.

All of these play directly into your hands – you're still playing a part of your passion, you're still in your niche.

MAXIMIZING YOUR SELF-ROI

You, as an individual, must be out to improve yourself as a business; that should be your top goal every day. This could be as simple as just reading a book, looking up a few websites, buying a hobby kit, signing up for a class, going back to school, or joining up with a mentor.

Expand, expand, expand. The more paths you explore, the more open doors for new pathways you'll find.

Know-It-A-Lot

If you go in with the mindset that you know everything there is to know already, you're not going to learn a single thing. The 'secret,' if there is one, is to strive to be the person who 'knows it all' – you don't just get one toe wet, or one foot, but put both feet in – and find your confidence in learning. This applies to every topic under the sun, from advanced cancer treatments and how viruses work all the way down to fixing a dishwasher or changing a tire. Home life, single or with a family, and work-life, nurse, student, or doctor, are intimately interconnected – one is not more important than the other.

In your smartphone, you have the opportunity to constantly learn something, to build on yourself and your future. Know something about a topic? Learn more. Do you know how chemotherapy works? Maybe so, but do you know what possible combinations of chemotherapy drugs are possible? Not as likely. How about a lasagna – do you know how to make one? What about a vegetarian version? Again, maybe, maybe not. Either way, the answers, now, in the digital age, are at your fingertips. There's no excuse not to explore the world that's been given to us.

That's maximizing our self-ROI.

Balancing Act

Without a balance, quite frankly, you'll drown in the ocean of possibilities and stresses of life. Everyone has a concept of a rigid schedule, especially in the middle world. After all, we've been through medical school, internships, and residencies! The problem is that once we're free and in the working world, a major portion of that rigid schedule slips away. Sure, we know we have to be at work for 8-10 hours a day, but what about the other hours?

Yes, you need a new scheduling system.

Are you going to exercise each day? You know you should. You've got to schedule in time with your family, sure...

What about time for learning and keeping your passions alive?

Keep Your Passion Burning

As an example, part of my own passion, as you've come to learn through the course of this book, is to provide my patients with certain procedures that could not be done at a hospital because of the costs associated with having them done there.

This is where the office-based surgery center doing cardiac catheterizations and revascularization came into play, cutting out all hospital fees and working a way in for my patients' copay to take care of the costs, being out of the traditional hospital environment, twisting the system a little, forcing the insurance system to do what it was built to do – protect clients' health. Can it be done cheaper in the clinic? Yes. Everyone wins.

Those simple tweaks made the biggest difference in the world.

That's what I wanted to do, to give my patients an opportunity to change their lives – at the deepest core of my passion for helping others, that's where the idea burned.

The Last Reminder

> *If you've learned only one thing from this book,*
> *then let it be this:*

Your self-worth is yourself. What you put in is equivalent to what you'll receive going out. Nothing less, nothing more. Keep your eyes open.

'It's hard to beat somebody who never gives up.'

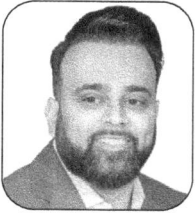

About Dr. Irfan Siddiqui

An Award-Winning Doctor and Entrepreneur, Dr. Irfan Siddiqui is a graduate of Nova Southeastern University College of Medicine. He graduated top of his class, followed by his Internal Medicine Residency and Cardiology Fellowship at Michigan State University. This was followed by a Specialty Fellowship of Interventional Cardiology at University of Utah, where he was part of national trials and registries. During his training, Dr Siddiqui was able to provide superior care along with leadership and was awarded Chief Resident and Chief Fellow positions. He provided great guidance and vision which paved the way for future doctors.

Dr Siddiqui has been practicing Interventional Cardiology for more than a decade and has been named TOP DOCTOR for multiple years. He has seen hundreds of thousands of patients and his compassion and surgical skills have changed the way the doctor-patient relationship is practiced.

He has multiple research trials, registries, and publications, the latest of which transformed the way Atrial Septal Defect surgeries are performed in the cardiac catheterization operating room. His procedural technique is used throughout the nation as a primary method minimizing radiation exposure.

Dr. Siddiqui is Triple Board Certified, including the specialties of Internal Medicine, Cardiology, and Interventional Cardiology. He has been acknowledged and awarded various other certifications and appointments. He is also an associate professor for local medical schools, nursing schools and colleges.

Dr. Siddiqui is a leader and visionary for The Business of Medicine. His vision of Health and Business has changed the way medicine is practiced on local to government levels. He founded the Private Insurance Operating Cardiac Model and the Time Share Cardiac Suite Concept, both of which systems are used nationally. His business was awarded TOP business of the year and his applications and ideas have trailblazed the way entrepreneurial medicine is practiced.

He has truly pioneered the way medicine is practiced on a Doctor-

Patient level and Doctor-Business Model. Yet another attribute was his Doctor Leaseback Program, which helped many physicians improve their businesses and financial standing.

Dr. Siddiqui is active in the community and enjoys traveling, playing poker and spending time with his wife Natalie, children Sameer and Maya...and their dog Bella.

Learn more at:
- www.drirfansiddiqui.com